ALCOHOL AND DRUG ABUSE

# OPIOID USE AND MISUSE IN THE MEDICARE SYSTEM

# Alcohol and Drug Abuse

Additional books and e-books in this series can be found on Nova's website under the Series tab.

ALCOHOL AND DRUG ABUSE

# OPIOID USE AND MISUSE IN THE MEDICARE SYSTEM

TOM FREITAG
EDITOR

snova
New York

## Library of Congress Cataloging-in-Publication Data

ISBN: 978-1-53616-858-7

*Published by Nova Science Publishers, Inc. † New York*

# CONTENTS


| | | |
|---|---|---|
| **Preface** | | **vii** |
| **Chapter 1** | Opioid Screening and Chronic Pain Management Alternatives for Seniors Act<br>*Committee on Energy and Commerce* | **1** |
| **Chapter 2** | Advancing High Quality Treatment for Opioid Use Disorders in Medicare Act<br>*Committee on Energy and Commerce* | **131** |
| **Chapter 3** | Strengthening Partnerships to Prevent Opioid Abuse Act<br>*Committee on Energy and Commerce* | **179** |
| **Index** | | **283** |
| **Related Nova Publications** | | **291** |

# PREFACE

The Medicare program serves as the healthcare coverage provider to over 58 million beneficiaries. In serving the over age 65 population, Medicare accounts for a large share of total opioid prescriptions. In 2016, one out of every three beneficiaries was prescribed an opioid through Medicare Part D. While many Medicare beneficiaries with serious pain-related conditions are being properly prescribed opioids, there is mounting evidence of opioid misuse in the Medicare system. This book looks at a proposed programs which seek to increase screening and thus, early detection of potential opioid use disorder upon entry into the Medicare program.

Chapter 1 - This is an edited, reformatted and augmented version of House of Representatives, 115th Congress, 2d Session, Publication No. Rept. 115–739; Part 1, dated JUNE 12, 2018.

Chapter 2 - This is an edited, reformatted and augmented version of House of Representatives Report, Committed to the Committee of the Whole House on the State of the Union and ordered to be printed, Publication No. 115–744, Part 1, dated June 12, 2018. H.R. 5605, Advancing High Quality Treatment for Opioid Use Disorders in Medicare, was introduced on April 24, 2018, by Rep. Raul Ruiz (D–CA), to create a demonstration project to test new ways to treat opioid use disorder among the Medicare population. This model includes the development of measures to evaluate the quality and outcomes of treatment.

Chapter 3 - This is an edited, reformatted and augmented version of House of Representatives 115th Congress, 2d Session, REPT. 115–737, Part 1, dated June 12, 2018.

In: Opioid Use and Misuse …
Editor: Tom Freitag

ISBN: 978-1-53616-858-7


*Chapter 1*

# OPIOID SCREENING AND CHRONIC PAIN MANAGEMENT ALTERNATIVES FOR SENIORS ACT*

***Committee on Energy and Commerce***

Mr. Walden, from the Committee on Energy and Commerce, submitted the following report [To accompany H.R. 5798]

[Including cost estimate of the Congressional Budget Office]

The Committee on Energy and Commerce, to whom was referred the bill (H.R. 5798) to amend title XVIII of the Social Security Act to require a review of current opioid prescriptions for chronic pain and screening for opioid use disorder to be included in the Welcome to Medicare initial preventive physical examination, having considered the same, report favorably thereon without amendment and recommend that the bill do pass.

* This is an edited, reformatted and augmented version of House of Representatives, 115th Congress, 2d Session, Publication No. Rept. 115–739; Part 1, dated JUNE 12, 2018.

## PURPOSE AND SUMMARY

H.R. 5798, Opioid Screening and Chronic Pain Management Alternatives for Seniors Act, was introduced on May 15, 2018, by Rep. Larry Bucshon (R–IN), Rep. Debbie Dingell (D–MI), and Rep. Erik Paulsen (R–MN) to add a review of current opioid prescriptions, a pain assessment, and, as appropriate, a screening for opioid use disorder as part of the Welcome to Medicare initial examination.

## BACKGROUND AND NEED FOR LEGISLATION

The Medicare program serves as the healthcare coverage provider to over 58 million beneficiaries. This number is projected to rise to over 80 million by 2030. In serving the over age 65 population, Medicare accounts for a large share of total opioid prescriptions. In 2016, one out of every three beneficiaries was prescribed an opioid through Medicare Part D. In total, this equates to almost 80 million prescriptions and $4 billion in Medicare Part D spending. While many Medicare beneficiaries with serious pain-related conditions are being properly prescribed opioids, there is mounting evidence of opioid misuse in the Medicare system. As more seniors and individuals with disabilities come into the program, the challenges of fraud, misuse, and abuse will only increase.

This bill seeks to increase screening and thus, early detection of potential opioid use disorder is addressed upon entry into the Medicare program. In the case of a beneficiary with a current opioid prescription for chronic pain, the bill requires qualified practitioners to review the beneficiary's potential risk factors for opioid use disorder, evaluate the beneficiary's level of pain, provide the beneficiary with information regarding non-opioid treatment options, and provide a referral for additional treatment, where appropriate.

## Committee Action

On April 11 and 12, 2018, the Subcommittee on Health held a hearing entitled "Combating the Opioid Crisis: Improving the Ability of Medicare and Medicaid to Provide Care for Patients" to review legislation related to the opioid epidemic. The Subcommittee received testimony from:

- Kimberly Brandt, Principal Deputy Administrator for Operations, Centers for Medicare and Medicaid Services, U.S. Department of Health and Human Services;
- Michael Botticelli, Executive Director, Grayken Center for Addiction, Boston Medical Center;
- Toby Douglas, Senior Vice President, Medicaid Solutions, Centene Corporation;
- David Guth, CEO, Centerstone;
- John Kravitz, CIO, Geisinger Health System; and,
- Sam Srivastava, CEO, Magellan Health.

On April 25, 2018, the Subcommittee on Health met in open markup session and forwarded a discussion draft, entitled "Welcome to Medicare," without amendment, to the full Committee by a voice vote. On May 17, 2018, the full Committee on Energy and Commerce met in open markup session and ordered H.R. 5798, without amendment, reported to the House by a voice vote. H.R. 5798 was similar to the discussion draft forwarded by the Subcommittee.

## Committee Votes

Clause 3(b) of rule XIII requires the Committee to list the record votes on the motion to report legislation and amendments thereto. There were no record votes taken in connection with ordering H.R. 5798 reported.

## OVERSIGHT FINDINGS AND RECOMMENDATIONS

Pursuant to clause 2(b)(1) of rule X and clause 3(c)(1) of rule XIII, the Committee held a hearing and made findings that are reflected in this report.

## NEW BUDGET AUTHORITY, ENTITLEMENT AUTHORITY, AND TAX EXPENDITURES

Pursuant to clause 3(c)(2) of rule XIII, the Committee finds that H.R. 5798 would result in no new or increased budget authority, entitlement authority, or tax expenditures or revenues.

## CONGRESSIONAL BUDGET OFFICE ESTIMATE

Pursuant to clause 3(c)(3) of rule XIII, the following is the cost estimate provided by the Congressional Budget Office pursuant to section 402 of the Congressional Budget Act of 1974:

U.S. Congress, Congressional Budget Office,
*Washington, DC, June 6, 2018.*

Hon. Greg Walden,
*Chairman, Committee on Energy and Commerce,*
*House of Representatives, Washington, DC.*

Dear Mr. Chairman: The Congressional Budget Office has prepared the enclosed document with cost estimates for the opioid-related legislation ordered to be reported on May 9 and May 17, 2018.

If you wish further details on this estimate, we will be pleased to provide them. The CBO staff contacts are Tom Bradley and Chad Chirico.

Sincerely,

Mark P. Hadley
(For Keith Hall, Director).

## Opioid Legislation

Summary: On May 9 and May 17, 2018, the House Committee on Energy and Commerce ordered 59 bills to be reported related to the nation's response to the opioid epidemic. Generally, the bills would:

- Provide grants to facilities and providers that treat people with substance use disorders,
- Direct various agencies within the Department of Health and Human Services (HHS) to explore nonopioid approaches to treating pain and to educate providers about those alternatives,
- Modify requirements under Medicaid and Medicare for prescribing controlled substances,
- Expand Medicaid coverage for substance abuse treatment, and
- Direct the Food and Drug Administration (FDA) to modify its oversight of opioid drugs and other medications that are used to manage pain.

Because of the large number of related bills ordered reported by the Committee, CBO is publishing a single comprehensive document that includes estimates for each piece of legislation.

CBO estimates that enacting 20 of the bills would affect direct spending, and 2 of the bills would affect revenues; therefore, pay-as-you-go procedures apply for those bills.

CBO estimates that enacting H.R. 4998, the Health Insurance for Former Foster Youth Act, would increase net direct spending by more than $2.5 billion and on-budget deficits by more than $5 billion in at least one of the four consecutive 10-year periods beginning in 2029.

None of the remaining 58 bills included in this estimate would increase net direct spending by more than $2.5 billion or on-budget deficits by more than $5 billion in any of the four consecutive 10-year periods beginning in 2029.

One of the bills reviewed for this document, H.R. 5795, would impose both intergovernmental and private-sector mandates as defined in the Unfunded Mandates Reform Act (UMRA). CBO estimates that the costs of those mandates on public and private entities would fall below the thresholds in UMRA ($80 million and $160 million, respectively, in 2018, adjusted annually for inflation). Five bills, H.R. 5228, H.R. 5333, H.R. 5554, H.R. 5687, and H.R. 5811, would impose private-sector mandates as defined in UMRA. CBO estimates that the costs of the mandates in three of the bills (H.R. 5333, H.R. 5554, and H.R. 5811) would not exceed the UMRA threshold for private entities. Because CBO is uncertain how federal agencies would implement new authority granted in the other two bills, H.R. 5228 and H.R. 5687, CBO cannot determine whether the costs of those mandates would exceed the UMRA threshold.

Estimated cost to the Federal Government: The estimates in this document do not include the effects of interactions among the bills. If all 59 bills were combined and enacted as one piece of legislation, the budgetary effects would be different from the sum of the estimates in this document, although CBO expects that any such differences would be small. The costs of this legislation fall within budget functions 550 (health), 570 (Medicare), 750 (administration of justice), and 800 (general government).

Basis of estimate: For this estimate, CBO assumes that all of the legislation will be enacted late in 2018 and that authorized and estimated amounts will be appropriated each year. Outlays for discretionary programs are estimated based on historical spending patterns for similar programs.

## Uncertainty

CBO aims to produce estimates that generally reflect the middle of a range of the most likely budgetary outcomes that would result if the legislation was enacted. Because data on the utilization of mental health and substance abuse treatment under Medicaid and Medicare is scarce, CBO cannot precisely predict how patients or providers would respond to some policy changes or what budgetary effects would result. In addition, several of the bills would give the Department of Health and Human Services (HHS) considerable latitude in designing and implementing policies. Budgetary effects could differ from those provided in CBO's analyses depending on those decisions.

## Direct Spending and Revenues

Table 1 lists the 22 bills of the 59 ordered to be reported that would affect direct spending or revenues.

Legislation Primarily Affecting Medicaid. The following nine bills would affect direct spending for the Medicaid program.

*H.R. 1925, the At-Risk Youth Medicaid Protection Act of 2017,* would require states to suspend, rather than terminate, Medicaid eligibility for juvenile enrollees (generally under 21 years of age) who become inmates of public correctional institutions. States also would have to redetermine those enrollees' Medicaid eligibility before their release and restore their coverage upon release if they qualify for the program. States would be required to process Medicaid applications submitted by or on behalf of juveniles in public correctional institutions who were not enrolled in Medicaid before becoming inmates and ensure that Medicaid coverage is provided when they are released if they are found to be eligible. On the basis of an analysis of juvenile incarceration trends and of the per enrollee spending for Medicaid foster care children, who have a similar health profile to incarcerated juveniles, CBO estimates that implementing the bill would cost $75 million over the 2019–2028 period.

## Table 1. Estimated Changes in Mandatory Spending and Revenues

| | By fiscal year, in millions of dollars— | | | | | | | | | | | | |
|---|---|---|---|---|---|---|---|---|---|---|---|---|---|
| | 2018 | 2019 | 2020 | 2021 | 2022 | 2023 | 2024 | 2025 | 2026 | 2027 | 2028 | 2019–2023 | 2019–2028 |
| | INCREASES OR DECREASES (-) IN DIRECT SPENDING | | | | | | | | | | | | |
| Legislation Primarily Affecting Medicaid: | | | | | | | | | | | | | |
| H.R. 1925, At-Risk Youth Medicaid Protection Act of 2017 | 0 | * | 5 | 5 | 5 | 10 | 10 | 10 | 10 | 10 | 10 | 25 | 75 |
| H.R. 4998, Health Insurance for Former Foster Youth Act | 0 | 0 | 0 | 0 | 0 | * | 10 | 21 | 33 | 46 | 61 | * | 171 |
| H.R. 5477, Rural Development of Opioid Capacity Services Act | 0 | 13 | 35 | 58 | 68 | 83 | 27 | 9 | 3 | 3 | 3 | 256 | 301 |
| H.R. 5583, a bill to amend title XI of the Social Security Act to require States to annually report on certain adult health quality measures, and for other purposes | 0 | * | * | * | * | * | * | * | * | * | * | * | * |
| H.R. 5797, IMD CARE Act | 0 | 38 | 158 | 251 | 265 | 279 | 0 | 0 | 0 | 0 | 0 | 991 | 991 |
| H.R. 5799, Medicaid DRUG Improvement Act[a] | 0 | * | * | 1 | 1 | 1 | 1 | 1 | 1 | 1 | 1 | 2 | 5 |
| H.R. 5801 Medicaid Providers Are Required To Note Experiences in Record Systems to Help In-Need Patients (PARTNERSHIP) Act[a] | 0 | * | * | * | * | * | * | * | * | * | * | * | * |
| H.R. 5808, Medicaid Pharmaceutical Home Act of 2018[a] | 0 | * | -1 | -1 | -1 | -1 | -2 | -2 | -2 | -2 | -2 | -4 | -13 |
| H.R. 5810, Medicaid Health HOME Act | 0 | 94 | 58 | 62 | 56 | 52 | 48 | 43 | 38 | 32 | 25 | 323 | 509 |

| | By fiscal year, in millions of dollars— | | | | | | | | | | | | |
|---|---|---|---|---|---|---|---|---|---|---|---|---|---|
| | 2018 | 2019 | 2020 | 2021 | 2022 | 2023 | 2024 | 2025 | 2026 | 2027 | 2028 | 2019–2023 | 2019–2028 |
| Legislation Primarily Affecting Medicare: | | | | | | | | | | | | | |
| H.R. 3528, Every Prescription Conveyed Securely Act | 0 | 0 | 0 | -24 | -35 | -33 | -30 | -33 | -32 | -31 | -32 | -92 | -250 |
| H.R. 4841, Standardizing Electronic Prior Authorization for Safe Prescribing Act of 2018 | 0 | 0 | 0 | * | * | * | * | * | * | * | * | * | * |
| H.R. 5603, Access to Telehealth Services for Opioid Use Disorders Act | 0 | 2 | * | * | * | 1 | 1 | 1 | 2 | 2 | 2 | 3 | 11 |
| H.R. 5605, Advancing High Quality Treatment for Opioid Use Disorders in Medicare Act | 0 | 0 | 0 | 15 | 26 | 24 | 23 | 23 | 10 | 1 | * | 65 | 122 |
| H.R. 5675, a bill to amend title XVIII of the Social Security Act to require prescription drug plan sponsors under the Medicare program to establish drug management programs for at-risk beneficiaries | 0 | 0 | 0 | -6 | -7 | -7 | -7 | -8 | -9 | -9 | -11 | -20 | -64 |
| H.R. 5684, Protecting Seniors From Opioid Abuse Act | 0 | 0 | 0 | * | * | * | * | * | * | * | * | * | * |
| H.R. 5796, Responsible Education Achieves Care and Healthy Outcomes for Users' Treatment Act of 2018 | 0 | 10 | 25 | 50 | 10 | 5 | 0 | 0 | 0 | 0 | 0 | 100 | 100 |
| H.R. 5798, Opioid Screening and Chronic Pain Management Alternatives for Seniors Act. | 0 | 0 | * | 1 | 1 | 1 | 1 | 1 | 1 | 1 | 1 | 2 | 5 |

**Table 1. (Continued)**

| | By fiscal year, in millions of dollars— | | | | | | | | | | | | |
|---|---|---|---|---|---|---|---|---|---|---|---|---|---|
| | 2018 | 2019 | 2020 | 2021 | 2022 | 2023 | 2024 | 2025 | 2026 | 2027 | 2028 | 2019–2023 | 2019–2028 |
| H.R. 5804, Post-Surgical Injections as an Opioid Alternative Act[a] | 0 | 0 | 25 | 30 | 25 | 20 | 10 | 5 | 0 | 0 | 0 | 100 | 115 |
| H.R. 5809, Postoperative Opioid Prevention Act of 2018 | 0 | 0 | 0 | 0 | 10 | 15 | 20 | 25 | 30 | 35 | 45 | 25 | 180 |
| Legislation Primarily Affecting the Food and Drug Administration: | | | | | | | | | | | | | |
| H.R. 5333, Over-the-Counter Monograph Safety, Innovation, and Reform Act of 2018[a] | 0 | 0 | * | * | * | * | * | * | * | * | * | * | * |
| Increases Or Decreases (-) in Revenues[b] | | | | | | | | | | | | | |
| H.R. 5752, Stop Illicit Drug Importation Act of 2018 | 0 | * | * | * | * | * | * | * | * | * | * | * | * |

Annual amounts may not sum to totals because of rounding. * = between -$500,000 and $500,000. Budget authority is equivalent to outlays.

[a] This bill also would affect spending subject to appropriation.

[b] One additional bill, H.R. 5228, the Stop Counterfeit Drugs by Regulating and Enhancing Enforcement Now Act, would have a negligible effect on revenues.

*H.R. 4998, the Health Insurance for Former Foster Youth Act,* would require states to provide Medicaid coverage to adults up to age 25 who had aged out of foster care in any state. Under current law, such coverage is mandatory only if the former foster care youth has aged out in the state in which the individual applies for coverage. The policy also would apply to former foster children who had been in foster care upon turning 14 years of age but subsequently left foster care to enter into a legal guardianship with a kinship caregiver. The provisions would take effect respect for foster youth who turn 18 on or after January 1, 2023. On the basis of spending for Medicaid foster care children and data from the Census Bureau regarding annual migration rates between states, CBO estimates that implementing the bill would cost $171 million over the 2019–2028 period.

*H.R. 5477, the Rural Development of Opioid Capacity Services Act,* would direct the Secretary of HHS to conduct a five-year demonstration to increase the number and ability of providers participating in Medicaid to provide treatment for substance use disorders. On the basis of an analysis of federal and state spending for treatment of substance use disorders and the prevalence of such disorders, CBO estimates that enacting the bill would increase direct spending by $301 million over the 2019–2028 period.

*H.R. 5583, a bill to amend title XI of the Social Security Act to require States to annually report on certain adult health quality measures, and for other purposes,* would require states to include behavioral health indicators in their annual reports on the quality of care under Medicaid. Although the bill would add a requirement for states, CBO estimates that its enactment would not have a significant budgetary effect because most states have systems in place for reporting such measures to the federal government.

*H.R. 5797, the IMD CARE Act,* would expand Medicaid coverage for people with opioid use disorder who are in institutions for mental disease (IMDs) for up to 30 days per year. Under a current-law policy known as the IMD exclusion, the federal government generally does not make matching payments to state Medicaid programs for most services provided by IMDs to adults between the ages of 21 and 64. Recent administrative changes have made federal financing for IMDs available in limited circumstances, but the statutory prohibition remains in place. CBO analyzed several data sets, primarily those collected by the Substance Abuse and Mental Health Services Administration (SAMHSA), to estimate current federal spending under Medicaid for IMD services and to estimate spending under H.R. 5797. Using that analysis, CBO estimates that enacting H.R. 5797 would increase direct spending by $991 million over the 2019–2028 period.

*H.R. 5799, the Medicaid DRUG Improvement Act,* would require state Medicaid programs to implement additional reviews of opioid prescriptions, monitor concurrent prescribing of opioids and certain other drugs, and monitor use of antipsychotic drugs by children. CBO estimates that the bill would increase direct spending by $5 million over 2019–2028 period to cover the administrative costs of complying with those requirements. On the basis of stakeholder feedback, CBO expects that the bill would not have a significant effect on Medicaid spending for prescription drugs because many of the bill's requirements would duplicate current efforts to curb opioid and antipsychotic drug use. (If enacted, H.R. 5799 also would affect spending subject to appropriation; CBO has not completed an estimate of that amount.)

*H.R. 5801, the Medicaid Providers Are Required To Note Experiences in Record Systems to Help-In-Need Patients (PARTNERSHIP) Act,* would require providers who are permitted to prescribe controlled substances and who participate in Medicaid to query prescription drug monitoring programs (PDMPs) before prescribing controlled substances to Medicaid patients. PDMPs are statewide electronic databases that collect data on controlled substances dispensed in the state. The bill also would require PDMPs to comply with certain data and system criteria, and it would provide additional federal matching funds to certain states to help cover administrative costs. On the basis of a literature review and stakeholder feedback, CBO estimates that the net budgetary effect of enacting H.R. 5801 would be insignificant. Costs for states to come into compliance with the systems and administrative requirements would be roughly offset by savings from small reductions in the number of controlled substances paid for by Medicaid under the proposal. (If enacted, H.R. 5801 also would affect spending subject to appropriation; CBO has not completed an estimate of that amount.)

*H.R. 5808, the Medicaid Pharmaceutical Home Act of 2018,* would require state Medicaid programs to operate pharmacy programs that would identify people at high risk of abusing controlled substances and require those patients to use a limited number of providers and pharmacies. Although nearly all state Medicaid programs currently meet such a requirement, a small number of high-risk Medicaid beneficiaries are not now monitored. Based on an analysis of information about similar state and federal programs, CBO estimates that net Medicaid spending under the bill would decrease by $13 million over the 2019–2028 period. That amount represents a small increase in administrative costs and a small reduction in the number of controlled substances paid for by Medicaid under the proposal. (If enacted, H.R. 5808 also would affect spending subject to appropriation; CBO has not completed an estimate of that amount.)

*H.R. 5810, the Medicaid Health HOME Act,* would allow states to receive six months of enhanced federal Medicaid funding for programs that coordinate care for people with substance use disorders. Based on enrollment and spending data from states that currently participate in Medicaid's Health Homes program, CBO estimates that the expansion would cost approximately $469 million over the 2019–2028 period. The bill also would require states to cover all FDA-approved drugs used in medication-assisted treatment for five years, although states could seek a waiver from that requirement. (Medication-assisted treatment combines behavioral therapy and pharmaceutical treatment for substance use disorders.) Under current law, states already cover most FDA-approved drugs used in such programs in some capacity, although a few exclude methadone dispensed by opioid treatment programs. CBO estimates that a small share of those states would begin to cover methadone if this bill was enacted at a federal cost of about $39 million over the 2019–2028 period. In sum, CBO estimates that the enacting H.R. 5810 would increase direct spending by $509 million over the 2019–2028 period.

Legislation Primarily Affecting Medicare. The following ten bills would affect direct spending for the Medicare program.

*H.R. 3528, the Every Prescription Conveyed Securely Act,* would require prescriptions for controlled substances covered under Medicare Part D to be transmitted electronically, starting on January 1, 2021. Based on CBO's analysis of prescription drug spending, spending for controlled substances is a small share of total drug spending. CBO also assumes a small share of those prescriptions would not be filled because they are not converted to an electronic format. Therefore, CBO expects that enacting H.R. 3528 would reduce the number of prescriptions filled and estimates that Medicare spending would be reduced by $250 million over the 2019–2028 period.

*H.R. 4841, the Standardizing Electronic Prior Authorization for Safe Prescribing Act of 2018,* would require health care professionals to submit prior authorization requests electronically, starting on January 1, 2021, for drugs covered under Medicare Part D. Taking into account that many prescribers already use electronic methods to submit such requests, CBO estimates that enacting H.R. 4841 would not significantly affect direct spending for Part D.

*H.R. 5603, the Access to Telehealth Services for Opioid Use Disorders Act,* would permit the Secretary of HHS to lift current geographic and other restrictions on coverage of telehealth services under Medicare for treatment of substance use disorders or co-occurring mental health disorders. Under the bill, the Secretary of HHS would be directed to encourage other payers to coordinate payments for opioid use disorder treatments and to evaluate the extent to which the demonstration reduces hospitalizations, increases the use of medication-assisted treatments, and improves the health outcomes of individuals with opioid use disorders during and after the demonstration. Based on current use of Medicare telehealth services for treatment of substance use disorders, CBO estimates that expanding that coverage would increase direct spending by $11 million over the 2019–2028 period.

*H.R. 5605, the Advancing High Quality Treatment for Opioid Use Disorders in Medicare Act,* would establish a five-year demonstration program to increase access to treatment for opioid use disorder. The demonstration would provide incentive payments and funding for care management services based on criteria such as patient engagement, use of evidence-based treatments, and treatment length and intensity. Under the bill, the Secretary of HHS would be directed to encourage other payers to coordinate payments for opioid use disorder treatments and to evaluate the extent to which the demonstration reduces hospitalizations, increases the use of medication-assisted treatments, and improves the health outcomes of individuals with opioid use disorders during and after the demonstration. Based on historical utilization of opioid use disorder treatments and projected spending on incentive payments and care management fees, CBO estimates that increased use of treatment services and the demonstration's incentive payments would increase direct spending by $122 million over the 2019–2028 period.

*H.R. 5675, a bill to amend title XVIII of the Social Security Act to require prescription drug plan sponsors under the Medicare program to establish drug management programs for at-risk beneficiaries,* would require Part D prescription drug plans to provide drug management programs for Medicare beneficiaries who are at risk for prescription drug abuse. (Under current law, Part D plans are permitted but not required to establish such programs as of 2019.) Based on an analysis of the number of plans currently providing those programs, CBO estimates that enacting H.R. 5675 would lower federal spending by $64 million over the 2019–2028 period by reducing the number of prescriptions filled and Medicare's payments for controlled substances.

*H.R. 5684, the Protecting Seniors From Opioid Abuse Act,* would expand medication therapy management programs under Medicare Part D to include beneficiaries who are at risk for prescription drug abuse. Because relatively few beneficiaries would be affected by this bill, CBO estimates that its enactment would not significantly affect direct spending for Part D.

*H.R. 5796, the Responsible Education Achieves Care and Healthy Outcomes for Users' Treatment Act of 2018,* would allow the Secretary of HHS to award grants to certain organizations that provide technical assistance and education to high-volume prescribers of opioids. The bill would appropriate $100 million for fiscal year 2019. Based on historical spending patterns for similar activities, CBO estimates that implementing H.R. 5796 would cost $100 million over the 2019–2028 period.

*H.R. 5798, the Opioid Screening and Chronic Pain Management Alternatives for Seniors Act,* would add an assessment of current opioid prescriptions and screening for opioid use disorder to the Welcome to Medicare Initial Preventive Physical Examination. Based on historical use of the examinations and pain management alternatives, CBO expects that enacting the bill would increase use of pain management services and estimates that direct spending would increase by $5 million over the 2019–2028 period.

*H.R. 5804, the Post-Surgical Injections as an Opioid Alternative Act,* would freeze the Medicare payment rate for certain analgesic injections provided in ambulatory surgical centers (ASCs). (For injections identified by specific billing codes, Medicare would pay the 2016 rate, which is higher than the current rate, during the 2020–2024 period.) Based on current utilization in the ASC setting, CBO estimates that enacting the legislation would increase direct spending by about $115 million over the 2019–2028 period. (If enacted,

H.R. 5804 also would affect spending subject to appropriation; see Table 3.)

*H.R. 5809, the Postoperative Opioid Prevention Act of 2018,* would create an additional payment under Medicare for nonopioid analgesics. Under current law, certain new drugs and devices may receive an additional payment—separate from the bundled payment for a surgical procedure—in outpatient hospital departments and ambulatory surgical centers. The bill would allow nonopioid analgesics to qualify for a five-year period of additional payments. Based on its assessment of current spending for analgesics and on the probability of new nonopioid analgesics coming to market, CBO estimates that H.R. 5809 would increase direct spending by about $180 million over the 2019–2028 period.

Legislation Primarily Affecting the Food and Drug Administration. One bill related to the FDA would affect direct spending.

*H.R. 5333, the Over-the-Counter Monograph Safety, Innovation, and Reform Act of 2018,* would change the way that the FDA regulates the marketing of over-the-counter (OTC) medicines, and it would authorize that agency to grant 18 months of exclusive market protection for certain qualifying OTC drugs, thus delaying the entry of other versions of the same qualifying OTC product. Medicaid currently provides some coverage for OTC medicines, but only if a medicine is the least costly alternative in its drug class. On the basis of stakeholder feedback, CBO expects that delaying the availability of additional OTC versions of a drug would not significantly affect the average net price paid by Medicaid. As a result, CBO estimates that enacting H.R. 5333 would have a negligible effect on the federal budget. (If enacted, H.R. 5333 also would affect spending subject to appropriation; see Table 3).

Legislation with Revenue Effects. Two bills would affect revenues. However, CBO estimates that one bill, H.R. 5228, the Stop Counterfeit Drugs by Regulating and Enhancing Enforcement Now Act, would have only a negligible effect.

*H.R. 5752, the Stop Illicit Drug Importation Act of 2018,* would amend the Federal, Food, Drug, and Cosmetic Act (FDCA) to strengthen the FDA's seizure powers and enhance its authority to detain, refuse, seize, or destroy illegal products offered for import. The legislation would subject more people to debarment under the FDCA and thus increase the potential for violations, and subsequently, the assessment of civil penalties, which are recorded in the budget as revenues. CBO estimates that those collections would result in an insignificant increase in revenues. Because H.R. 5752 would prohibit the importation of drugs that are in the process of being scheduled, it also could reduce amounts collected in customs duties. CBO anticipates that the result would be a negligible decrease in revenues. With those results taken together, CBO estimates, enacting H.R. 5752 would generate an insignificant net increase in revenues over the 2019–2028 period.

## Spending Subject to Appropriation

For this document, CBO has grouped bills with spending that would be subject to appropriation into four general categories:

- Bills that would have no budgetary effect,
- Bills with provisions that would authorize specified amounts to be appropriated (see Table 2),
- Bills with provisions for which CBO has estimated an authorization of appropriations (see Table 3), and
- Bills with provisions that would affect spending subject to appropriation for which CBO has not yet completed an estimate.

No Budgetary Effect. CBO estimates that 6 of the 59 bills would have no effect on direct spending, revenues, or spending subject to appropriation.

*H.R. 3192, the CHIP Mental Health Parity Act,* would require all Children's Health Insurance Program (CHIP) plans to cover mental health and substance abuse treatment. In addition, states would not be allowed to impose financial or utilization limits on mental health treatment that are lower than limits placed on physical health treatment. Based on information from the Centers for Medicare and Medicaid Services, CBO estimates that enacting the bill would have no budgetary effect because all CHIP enrollees are already in plans that meet those requirements.

*H.R. 3331, a bill to amend title XI of the Social Security Act to promote testing of incentive payments for behavioral health providers for adoption and use of certified electronic health record technology,* would give the Center for Medicare and Medicaid Innovation (CMMI) explicit authorization to test a program offering incentive payments to behavioral health providers that adopt and use certified electronic health record technology. Because it is already clear to CMMI that it has that authority, CBO estimates that enacting the legislation would not affect federal spending.

*H.R. 5202, the Ensuring Patient Access to Substance Use Disorder Treatments Act of 2018,* would clarify permission for pharmacists to deliver controlled substances to providers under certain circumstances. Because this provision would codify current practice, CBO estimates that H.R. 5202 would not affect direct spending or revenues during the 2019–2028 period.

*H.R. 5685, the Medicare Opioid Safety Education Act of 2018,* would require the Secretary of HHS to include information on opioid use, pain management, and nonopioid pain management treatments in future editions of *Medicare & You,* the program's handbook for beneficiaries, starting on January 1, 2019. Because H.R. 5685 would add information to an existing administrative document, CBO estimates that enacting the bill would have no budgetary effect.

*H.R. 5686, the Medicare Clear Health Options in Care for Enrollees Act of 2018,* would require prescription drug plans that provide coverage under Medicare Part D to furnish information to beneficiaries about the risks of opioid use and the availability of alternative treatments for pain. CBO estimates that enacting the bill would not affect direct spending because the required activities would not impose significant administrative costs.

*H.R. 5716, the Commit to Opioid Medical Prescriber Accountability and Safety for Seniors Act,* would require the Secretary of HHS on an annual basis to identify high prescribers of opioids and furnish them with information about proper prescribing methods. Because HHS already has the capacity to meet those requirements, CBO estimates that enacting that provision would not impose additional administrative costs on the agency.

Specified Authorizations. Table 2 lists the ten bills that would authorize specified amounts to be appropriated over the 2019–2023 period. Spending from those authorized amounts would be subject to appropriation.

**Table 2. Estimated spending subject to appropriation for bills with specified authorizations**

| | By fiscal year, in millions of dollars— | | | | | | |
|---|---|---|---|---|---|---|---|
| | **2018** | **2019** | **2020** | **2021** | **2022** | **2023** | **2019-2023** |
| Increases In Spending Subject To Appropriation | | | | | | | |
| H.R. 4684, Ensuring Access to Quality Sober Living Act: | | | | | | | |
| Authorization Level | 0 | 3 | 0 | 0 | 0 | 0 | 3 |
| Estimated Outlays | 0 | 1 | 2 | * | * | * | 3 |
| H.R. 5102, Substance Use Disorder Workforce Loan Repayment Act of 2018: | | | | | | | |
| Authorization Level | 0 | 25 | 25 | 25 | 25 | 25 | 125 |
| Estimated Outlays | 0 | 9 | 19 | 23 | 25 | 25 | 100 |
| H.R. 5176, Preventing Overdoses While in Emergency Rooms Act of 2018: | | | | | | | |
| Authorization Level | 0 | 50 | 0 | 0 | 0 | 0 | 50 |
| Estimated Outlays | 0 | 16 | 26 | 6 | 2 | 1 | 50 |
| H.R. 5197, Alternatives to Opioids (ALTO) in the Emergency Department Act: | | | | | | | |
| Authorization Level | 0 | 10 | 10 | 10 | 0 | 0 | 30 |
| Estimated Outlays | 0 | 3 | 8 | 10 | 7 | 2 | 30 |
| H.R. 5261, Treatment, Education, and Community Help to Combat Addiction Act of 2018: | | | | | | | |
| Authorization Level | 0 | 4 | 4 | 4 | 4 | 4 | 20 |
| Estimated Outlays | 0 | 1 | 3 | 4 | 4 | 4 | 16 |
| H.R. 5327, Comprehensive Opioid Recovery Centers Act of 2018: | | | | | | | |
| Authorization Level | 0 | 10 | 10 | 10 | 10 | 10 | 50 |
| Estimated Outlays | 0 | 3 | 8 | 10 | 10 | 10 | 41 |
| H.R. 5329, Poison Center Network Enhancement Act of 2018: | | | | | | | |
| Authorization Level | 0 | 30 | 30 | 30 | 30 | 30 | 151 |
| Estimated Outlays | 0 | 12 | 25 | 29 | 29 | 29 | 125 |
| H.R. 5353, Eliminating Opioid-Related Infectious Diseases Act of 2018: | | | | | | | |
| Authorization Level | 0 | 40 | 40 | 40 | 40 | 40 | 200 |
| Estimated Outlays. | 0 | 15 | 34 | 38 | 39 | 40 | 166 |
| H.R. 5580, Surveillance and Testing of Opioids to Prevent Fentanyl Deaths Act of 2018: | | | | | | | |
| Authorization Level | 30 | 30 | 30 | 30 | 30 | 0 | 120 |
| Estimated Outlays | 0 | 11 | 25 | 29 | 29 | 19 | 113 |
| H.R. 5587, Peer Support Communities of Recovery Act: | | | | | | | |
| Authorization Level | 0 | 15 | 15 | 15 | 15 | 15 | 75 |
| Estimated Outlays | 0 | 5 | 13 | 14 | 15 | 15 | 62 |

Annual amounts may not sum to totals because of rounding. * = between zero and $500,000.

*H.R. 4684, the Ensuring Access to Quality Sober Living Act,* would direct the Secretary of HHS to develop and disseminate best practices for organizations that operate housing designed for people recovering from substance use disorders. The bill would authorize a total of $3 million over the 2019–2021 period for that purpose. Based on historical spending patterns for similar activities, CBO estimates that implementing H.R. 4684 would cost $3 million over the 2019–2023 period.

*H.R. 5102, the Substance Use Disorder Workforce Loan Repayment Act of 2018,* would establish a loan repayment program for mental health professionals who practice in areas with few mental health providers or with high rates of death from overdose and would authorize $25 million per year over the 2019–2028 period for that purpose. Based on historical spending patterns for similar activities, CBO estimates that implementing H.R. 5102 would cost $100 million over the 2019–2023 period; the remaining amounts would be spent in years after 2023.

*H.R. 5176, the Preventing Overdoses While in Emergency Rooms Act of 2018,* would require the Secretary of HHS to develop protocols and a grant program for health care providers to address the needs of people who survive a drug overdose, and it would authorize $50 million in 2019 for that purpose. Based on historical spending patterns for similar activities, CBO estimates that implementing H.R. 5176 would cost $50 million over the 2019–2023 period.

*H.R. 5197, the Alternatives to Opioids (ALTO) in the Emergency Department Act,* would direct the Secretary of HHS to carry out a demonstration program for hospitals and emergency departments to develop alternative protocols for pain management that limit the use of opioids and would authorize $10 million annually in grants for fiscal years 2019 through 2021. Based on historical spending patterns for similar programs, CBO estimates that implementing H.R. 5197 would cost $30 million over the 2019–2023 period.

*H.R. 5261, the Treatment, Education, and Community Help to Combat Addiction Act of 2018,* would direct the Secretary of HHS to designate regional centers of excellence to improve the training of health professionals who treat substance use disorders. The bill would authorize $4 million annually for grants to those programs over the 2019–2023 period. Based on historical spending patterns for similar activities, CBO estimates that implementing H.R. 5261 would cost $16 million over the

2019–2023 period; the remaining amounts would be spent in years after 2023.

*H.R. 5327, the Comprehensive Opioid Recovery Centers Act of 2018,* would direct the Secretary of HHS to award grants to at least 10 providers that offer treatment services for people with opioid use disorder, and it would authorize $10 million per year over the 2019–2023 period for that purpose. Based on historical spending patterns for similar activities, CBO estimates that implementing H.R. 5327 would cost $41 million over the 2019–2023 period; the remaining amounts would be spent in years after 2023.

*H.R. 5329, the Poison Center Network Enhancement Act of 2018,* would reauthorize the poison control center toll-free number, national media campaign, and grant program under the Public Health Service Act. Among other actions, H.R. 5329 would increase the share of poison control center funding that could be provided by federal grants. The bill would authorize a total of about $30 million per year over the 2019–2023 period. Based on historical spending patterns for similar activities, CBO estimates that implementing H.R. 5329 would cost $125 million over the 2019–2023 period; the remaining amounts would be spent in years after 2023.

*H.R 5353, the Eliminating Opioid Related Infectious Diseases Act of 2018,* would amend the Public Health Service Act by broadening the focus of surveillance and education programs from preventing and treating hepatitis C virus to preventing and treating infections associated with injection drug use. It would authorize $40 million per year over 2019–2023 period for that purpose. Based on historical spending patterns for similar activities, CBO estimates that implementing H.R. 5353 would cost $166 million over the 2019– 2023 period; the remaining amounts would be spent in years after 2023.

*H.R. 5580, the Surveillance and Testing of Opioids to Prevent Fentanyl Deaths Act of 2018,* would establish a grant program for public health laboratories that conduct testing for fentanyl and other synthetic opioids. It also would direct the Centers for Disease Control and Prevention to expand its drug surveillance program, with a particular focus on collecting data on fentanyl. The bill would authorize a total of $30 million per year over the 2018–2022 period for those activities. Based on historical spending patterns for similar activities, CBO estimates that implementing H.R. 5580 would cost $113 million over the 2019–2023 period; the remaining amounts would be spent in years after 2023.

*H.R. 5587, Peer Support Communities of Recovery Act,* would direct the Secretary of HHS to award grants to nonprofit organizations that support community-based, peer-delivered support, including technical support for the establishment of recovery community organizations, independent, nonprofit groups led by people in recovery and their families. The bill would authorize $15 million per year for the 2019–2023 period. Based on historical spending patterns for similar activities, CBO estimates that implementing H.R. 5587 would cost $62 million over the 2019–2023 period; the remaining amounts would be spent in years after 2023.

Estimated Authorizations. Table 3 shows CBO's estimates of the appropriations that would be necessary to implement 19 of the bills. Spending would be subject to appropriation of those amounts.

*H.R. 449, the Synthetic Drug Awareness Act of 2018,* would require the Surgeon General to report to the Congress on the health effects of synthetic psychoactive drugs on children between the ages of 12 and 18. Based on spending patterns for similar activities, CBO estimates that implementing H.R. 449 would cost approximately $1 million over the 2019–2023 period.

*H.R. 4005, the Medicaid Reentry Act,* would direct the Secretary of HHS to convene a group of stakeholders to develop and report to the Congress on best practices for addressing issues related to health care faced by those returning from incarceration to their communities. The bill also would require the Secretary to issue a letter to state Medicaid directors about relevant demonstration projects. Based on an analysis of anticipated workload, CBO estimates that implementing H.R. 4005 would cost less than $500,000 over the 2018–2023 period.

*H.R. 4275, the Empowering Pharmacists in the Fight Against Opioid Abuse Act,* would require the Secretary of HHS to develop and disseminate materials for training pharmacists, health care practitioners, and the public about the circumstances under which a pharmacist may decline to fill a prescription. Based on historical spending patterns for similar activities,

CBO estimates that costs to the federal government for the development and distribution of those materials would not be significant.

**Table 3. Estimated spending subject to appropriation for bills with estimated authorizations**

| | By fiscal year, in millions of dollars— | | | | | | |
|---|---|---|---|---|---|---|---|
| | 2018 | 2019 | 2020 | 2021 | 2022 | 2023 | 2019-2023 |
| | Increases in Spending Subject to Appropriation | | | | | | |
| H.R. 449, Synthetic Drug Awareness Act of 2018: | | | | | | | |
| Estimated Authorization Level | 0 | * | * | * | 0 | 0 | 1 |
| Estimated Outlays | 0 | * | * | * | 0 | 0 | 1 |
| H.R. 4005, Medicaid Reentry Act: | | | | | | | |
| Estimated Authorization Level | * | * | 0 | 0 | 0 | 0 | * |
| Estimated Outlays | * | * | 0 | 0 | 0 | 0 | * |
| H.R. 4275, Empowering Pharmacists in the Fight Against Opioid Abuse Act: | | | | | | | |
| Estimated Authorization Level | 0 | * | * | * | * | * | * |
| Estimated Outlays. | 0 | * | * | * | * | * | * |
| H.R. 5009, Jessie's Law: | | | | | | | |
| Estimated Authorization Level | 0 | * | * | * | * | * | * |
| Estimated Outlays | 0 | * | * | * | * | * | * |
| H.R. 5041, Safe Disposal of Unused Medication Act: | | | | | | | |
| Estimated Authorization Level | 0 | * | * | * | * | * | * |
| Estimated Outlays | 0 | * | * | * | * | * | * |
| H.R. 5272, Reinforcing Evidence-Based Standards Under Law in Treating Substance Abuse Act of 2018: | | | | | | | |
| Estimated Authorization Level | 0 | 1 | 1 | 1 | 1 | 1 | 4 |
| Estimated Outlays | 0 | 1 | 1 | 1 | 1 | 1 | 4 |
| H.R. 5333, Over-the-Counter Monograph Safety, Innovation, and Reform Act of 2018:[a] | | | | | | | |
| Food and Drug Administration: | | | | | | | |
| Collections from fees: | | | | | | | |
| Estimated Authorization Level | 0 | -22 | -22 | -26 | -35 | -42 | -147 |
| Estimated Outlays | 0 | -22 | -22 | -26 | -35 | -42 | -147 |
| Spending of fees: | | | | | | | |
| Estimated Authorization Level | 0 | 22 | 22 | 26 | 35 | 42 | 147 |
| Estimated Outlays | 0 | 6 | 17 | 30 | 44 | 41 | 137 |
| Net effect on FDA: | | | | | | | |
| Estimated Authorization Level | 0 | 0 | 0 | 0 | 0 | 0 | 0 |
| Estimated Outlays | 0 | -17 | -6 | 4 | 9 | * | -10 |
| Government Accountability Office: | | | | | | | |
| Estimated Authorization Level | 0 | 0 | 0 | 0 | 0 | * | * |
| Estimated Outlays | 0 | 0 | 0 | 0 | 0 | * | * |

| | By fiscal year, in millions of dollars— | | | | | | |
|---|---|---|---|---|---|---|---|
| | **2018** | **2019** | **2020** | **2021** | **2022** | **2023** | **2019-2023** |
| Total, H.R. 5333: | | | | | | | |
| Estimated Authorization Level | 0 | 0 | 0 | 0 | 0 | * | * |
| Estimated Outlays | 0 | -17 | -6 | 4 | 9 | * | -10 |
| H.R. 5473, Better Pain Management Through Better Data Act of 2018: | | | | | | | |
| Estimated Authorization Level | 0 | * | * | * | * | 0 | 1 |
| Estimated Outlays | 0 | * | * | * | * | * | 1 |
| H.R. 5483, Special Registration for Telemedicine Clarification Act of 2018: | | | | | | | |
| Estimated Authorization Level | 0 | * | * | * | * | * | * |
| Estimated Outlays | 0 | * | * | * | * | * | * |
| H.R. 5554, Animal Drug and Animal Generic Drug User Fee Amendments of 2018: | | | | | | | |
| Collections from fees: | | | | | | | |
| Animal drug fees | 0 | -30 | -31 | -32 | -33 | -34 | -159 |
| Generic animal drug fees | 0 | -18 | -19 | -19 | -20 | -21 | -97 |
| Total, Estimated Authorization Level | 0 | -49 | -50 | -51 | -53 | -55 | -257 |
| Total, Estimated Outlays | 0 | -49 | -50 | -51 | -53 | -55 | -257 |
| Spending of fees: | | | | | | | |
| Animal drug fees | 0 | 30 | 31 | 32 | 33 | 34 | 159 |
| Generic animal drug fees | 0 | 18 | 19 | 19 | 20 | 21 | 97 |
| Total, Estimated Authorization Level | 0 | 49 | 50 | 51 | 53 | 53 | 257 |
| Total, Estimated Outlays | 0 | 39 | 47 | 51 | 52 | 54 | 243 |
| Net changes in fees: | | | | | | | |
| Estimated Authorization Level | 0 | 0 | 0 | 0 | 0 | 0 | 0 |
| Estimated Outlays | 0 | -10 | -3 | * | * | * | -14 |
| Other effects: | | | | | | | |
| Estimated Authorization Level | 0 | 3 | 1 | 1 | 1 | 1 | 6 |
| Estimated Outlays | 0 | 2 | 1 | 1 | 1 | 1 | 6 |
| Total, H.R. 5554: | | | | | | | |
| Estimated Authorization Level | 0 | 3 | 1 | 1 | 1 | 1 | 6 |
| Estimated Outlays | 0 | -8 | -2 | 1 | * | * | -8 |
| H.R. 5582, Abuse Deterrent Access Act of 2018: | | | | | | | |
| Estimated Authorization Level | 0 | 0 | * | 0 | 0 | 0 | * |
| Estimated Outlays | 0 | 0 | * | 0 | 0 | 0 | * |
| H.R. 5590, Opioid Addiction Action Plan Act: | | | | | | | |
| Estimated Authorization Level | * | * | * | * | * | * | 2 |
| Estimated Outlays | * | * | * | * | * | * | 2 |
| H.R. 5687, Securing Opioids and Unused Narcotics with Deliberate Disposal and Packaging Act of 2018: | | | | | | | |
| Estimated Authorization Level | 0 | * | * | * | * | * | * |
| Estimated Outlays | 0 | * | * | * | * | * | * |

**Table 3. (Continued)**

| | By fiscal year, in millions of dollars— | | | | | | |
|---|---|---|---|---|---|---|---|
| | **2018** | **2019** | **2020** | **2021** | **2022** | **2023** | **2019-2023** |
| H.R. 5715, Strengthening Partnerships to Prevent Opioid Abuse Act: | | | | | | | |
| Estimated Authorization Level | 0 | 2 | 2 | 2 | 2 | 2 | 9 |
| Estimated Outlays | 0 | 2 | 2 | 2 | 2 | 2 | 9 |
| H.R. 5789, a bill to require the Secretary of Health and Human Services to issue guidance to improve care for infants with neonatal abstinence syndrome and their mothers, and to require the Comptroller General of the United States to conduct a study on gaps in Medicaid coverage for pregnant and postpartum women with substance use disorder: | | | | | | | |
| Estimated Authorization Level | 0 | 2 | 0 | 0 | 0 | 0 | 2 |
| Estimated Outlays | 0 | 2 | 0 | 0 | 0 | 0 | 2 |
| H.R. 5795, Overdose Prevention and Patient Safety Act: | | | | | | | |
| Estimated Authorization Level | 0 | 1 | 0 | 0 | 0 | 0 | 1 |
| Estimated Outlays | 0 | 1 | 0 | 0 | 0 | 0 | 1 |
| H.R. 5800, Medicaid IMD ADDITIONAL INFO Act: | | | | | | | |
| Estimated Authorization Level | 0 | 1 | 0 | 0 | 0 | 0 | 1 |
| Estimated Outlays | 0 | * | * | 0 | 0 | 0 | 1 |
| H.R. 5804, Post-Surgical Injections as an Opioid Alternative Act:[a] | | | | | | | |
| Estimated Authorization Level | 0 | 0 | 0 | 0 | 1 | 1 | 1 |
| Estimated Outlays | 0 | 0 | 0 | 0 | 1 | 1 | 1 |
| H.R. 5811, a bill to amend the Federal Food, Drug, and Cosmetic Act with respect to postapproval study requirements for certain controlled substances, and for other purposes: | | | | | | | |
| Estimated Authorization Level | 0 | * | * | * | * | * | * |
| Estimated Outlays | 0 | * | * | * | * | * | * |

Annual amounts may not sum to totals because of rounding. * = between ¥$500,000 and $500,000.
[a] This bill also would affect mandatory spending (see Table 1).

H.R. 5009, Jessie's Law, would require HHS, in collaboration with outside experts, to develop best practices for displaying information about opioid use disorder in a patient's medical record. HHS also would be required to develop and disseminate written materials annually to health care providers about what disclosures could be made while still complying with federal laws that govern health care privacy. Based on spending patterns for similar activities, CBO estimates that implementing H.R. 5009 would have an insignificant effect on spending over the 2019–2023 period.

H.R. 5041, the Safe Disposal of Unused Medication Act, would require hospice programs to have written policies and procedures for the disposal of controlled substances after a patient's death. Certain licensed employees of hospice programs would be permitted to assist in the disposal of controlled substances that were lawfully dispensed. Using information from the Department of Justice (DOJ), CBO estimates that implementing the bill would cost less than $500,000 over the 2019–2023 period.

H.R. 5272, the Reinforcing Evidence-Based Standards Under Law in Treating Substance Abuse Act of 2018, would require the newly established National Mental Health and Substance Use Policy Laboratory to issue guidance to applicants for SAMHSA grants that support evidence-based practices. Using information from HHS about the historical cost of similar activities, CBO estimates that enacting this bill would cost approximately $4 million over the 2019–2023 period.

H.R. 5333, the Over-the-Counter Monograph Safety, Innovation, and Reform Act of 2018, would change the FDA's oversight of the commercial marketing of OTC medicines and authorize the collection and spending of fees through 2023 to cover the costs of expediting the FDA's administrative procedures for certain regulatory activities relating to OTC products. Under H.R. 5333, CBO estimates, the FDA would assess about $147 million in fees over the 2019–2023 period that could be collected and made available for obligation only to the extent and in the amounts provided in advance in appropriation acts. Because the FDA could spend those fees, CBO estimates that the estimated budget authority for collections and spending would offset each other exactly in each year, although CBO expects that spending initially would lag behind collections. Assuming appropriation action consistent with the bill, CBO estimates that implementing H.R. 5333 would reduce net discretionary outlays by $10 million over the 2019–2023 period, primarily because of that lag. The bill also would require the Government Accountability Office to study exclusive market protections for certain qualifying OTC drugs authorized by the bill—a provision that CBO estimates would cost less than $500,000. (If enacted, H.R. 5333 also would affect mandatory spending; see Table 1.)

H.R. 5473, the Better Pain Management Through Better Data Act of 2018, would require that the FDA conduct a public meeting and issue guidance to industry addressing data collection and labeling for medical products that reduce pain while enabling the reduction, replacement, or avoidance of oral opioids. Using information from the agency, CBO estimates that implementing H.R. 5473 would cost about $1 million over the 2019–2023 period.

H.R. 5483, the Special Registration for Telemedicine Clarification Act of 2018, would direct DOJ, within one year of the bill's enactment, to issue regulations concerning the practice of telemedicine (for remote diagnosis and treatment of patients). Using information from DOJ, CBO estimates that implementing the bill would cost less than $500,000 over the 2019–2023 period.

H.R. 5554, the Animal Drug and Animal Generic Drug User Fee Amendments of 2018, would authorize the FDA to collect and spend fees to cover the cost of expedited approval for the development and marketing of certain drugs for use in animals. The legislation would extend through fiscal year 2023, and make several changes to, the FDA's existing approval processes and fee programs for brand-name and generic veterinary drugs, which expire at the end of fiscal year 2018. CBO estimates that implementing H.R. 5554 would reduce net discretionary outlays by $8 million over the 2019–2023 period, primarily because the spending of fees lags somewhat behind their collection.

Fees authorized under the bill would supplement funds appropriated to cover the FDA's cost of reviewing certain applications and investigational submissions for brand-name and generic drugs for use in animals. Those fees could be collected and made available for obligation only to the extent and in the amounts provided in advance in appropriation acts. Under H.R. 5554, CBO estimates, the FDA would assess about $257 million in fees over the 2019–2023 period. Because the FDA could spend those funds, CBO estimates that budget authority for collections and spending would offset each other exactly in each year. CBO estimates that the delay between collecting and spending fees under the reauthorized programs would reduce net discretionary outlays by $14 million over the 2019–2023 period, assuming appropriation actions consistent with the bill.

Enacting H.R. 5554 would increase the FDA's workload because the legislation would expand eligibility for conditional approval for certain drugs. The agency's administrative costs also would increase because of regulatory activities required by a provision concerning petitions for additives intended for use in animal food. H.R. 5554 also would require the FDA to publish guidance or produce regulations on a range of topics, transmit a report to the Congress, and hold public meetings. CBO expects that the costs associated with those activities would not be covered by fees, and it estimates that implementing such provisions would cost $6 million over the 2019–2023 period.

H.R. 5582, the Abuse Deterrent Access Act of 2018, would require the Secretary of HHS to report to the Congress on existing barriers to access to "abuse-deterrent opioid formulations" by Medicare Part C and D beneficiaries. Such formulations make the drugs more difficult to dissolve for injection, for example, and thus can impede their abuse. Assuming the availability of appropriated funds and based on historical spending patterns for similar activities, CBO estimates that implementing the legislation would cost less than $500,000 over the 2019–2023 period.

H.R. 5590, the Opioid Addiction Action Plan Act, would require the Secretary of HHS to develop an action plan by January 1, 2019, for increasing access to medication-assisted treatment among Medicare and Medicaid enrollees. The bill also would require HHS to convene a stakeholder meeting and issue a request for information within three months of enactment, and to submit a report to the Congress by June 1, 2019. Based on historical spending patterns for similar activities, CBO estimates that implementing H.R. 5590 would cost approximately $2 million over the 2019–2023 period.

H.R. 5687, the Securing Opioids and Unused Narcotics with Deliberate Disposal and Packaging Act of 2018, would permit the FDA to require certain packaging and disposal technologies, controls, or measures to mitigate the risk of abuse and misuse of drugs. Based on information from the FDA, CBO estimates that implementing H.R. 5687 would not significantly affect spending over the 2019–2023 period. This bill would also require that the GAO study the effectiveness and use of packaging technologies for controlled substances—a provision that CBO estimates would cost less than $500,000.

H.R. 5715, the Strengthening Partnerships to Prevent Opioid Abuse Act, would require the Secretary of HHS to establish a secure Internet portal to allow HHS, Medicare Advantage plans, and Medicare Part D plans to exchange information about fraud, waste, and abuse among providers and suppliers no later than two years after enactment. H.R. 5715 also would require organizations with Medicare Advantage contracts to submit information on investigations related to providers suspected of prescribing large volumes of opioids through a process established by the Secretary no later than January 2021. Based on historical spending patterns for similar activities, CBO estimates that implementing H.R. 5715 would cost approximately $9 million over the 2019–2023 period.

H.R. 5789, a bill to require the Secretary of Health and Human Services to issue guidance to improve care for infants with neonatal abstinence syndrome and their mothers, and to require the Comptroller General of the United States to conduct a study on gaps in Medicaid coverage for pregnant and postpartum women with substance use disorder, would direct the Secretary of HHS to issue guidance to states on best practices under Medicaid and CHIP for treating infants with neonatal abstinence syndrome. H.R. 5789 also would direct the Government Accountability Office to study Medicaid coverage for pregnant and postpartum women with substance use disorders. Based on information from HHS and historical spending patterns for similar activities, CBO estimates that enacting H.R. 5789 would cost approximately $2 million over the 2019– 2023 period.

H.R. 5795, the Overdose Prevention and Patient Safety Act, would amend the Public Health Service Act so that requirements pertaining to the confidentiality and disclosure of medical records relating to substance use disorders align with the provisions of the Health Insurance Portability and Accountability Act of 1996. The bill would require the Office of the Secretary of HHS to issue regulations prohibiting discrimination based on data disclosed from such medical records, to issue regulations requiring covered entities to provide written notice of privacy practices, and to develop model training programs and materials for health care providers and patients and their families. Based on spending patterns for similar activities, CBO estimates that implementing H.R. 5795 would cost approximately $1 million over the 2019–2023 period.

H.R. 5800, Medicaid IMD ADDITIONAL INFO Act, would direct the Medicaid and CHIP Payment and Access Commission to study institutions for mental diseases in a representative sample of states. Based on information from the commission about the cost of similar work, CBO estimates that implementing H.R. 5800 would cost about $1 million over the 2019–2023 period.

H.R. 5804, the Post-Surgical Injections as an Opioid Alternative Act, would freeze the Medicare payment rate for certain analgesic injections provided in ambulatory surgical centers. The bill also would mandate two studies of Medicare coding and payments arising from enactment of this legislation. Based on the cost of similar activities, CBO estimates that those reports would cost $1 million over the 2019–2023 period. (If enacted, H.R. 5804 also would affect mandatory spending; see Table 1.)

H.R. 5811, a bill to amend the Federal Food, Drug, and Cosmetic Act with respect to postapproval study requirements for certain controlled substances, and for other purposes, would allow the FDA to require that pharmaceutical manufacturers study certain drugs after they are approved to assess any potential reduction in those drugs' effectiveness for the conditions of use prescribed, recommended, or suggested in labeling. CBO anticipates that implementing H.R. 5811 would not significantly affect the FDA's costs over the 2019–2023 period.

Other Authorizations. The following nine bills would increase authorization levels, but CBO has not completed estimates of amounts. All authorizations would be subject to future appropriation action.

- H.R. 4284, Indexing Narcotics, Fentanyl, and Opioids Act of 2017
- H.R. 5002, Advancing Cutting Edge Research Act
- H.R. 5228, Stop Counterfeit Drugs by Regulating and Enhancing Enforcement Now Act (see Table 1 for an estimate of the revenue effects of H.R. 5228)
- H.R. 5752, Stop Illicit Drug Importation Act of 2018 (see Table 1 for an estimate of the revenue effects of H.R. 5752)

- H.R. 5799, Medicaid DRUG Improvement Act (see Table 1 for an estimate of the direct spending effects of H.R. 5799)
- H.R. 5801, Medicaid Providers and Pharmacists Are Required to Note Experiences in Record Systems to Help In-Need Patients (PARTNERSHIP) Act (see Table 1 for an estimate of the direct spending effects of H.R. 5801)
- H.R. 5806, 21st Century Tools for Pain and Addiction Treatments Act
- H.R. 5808, Medicaid Pharmaceutical Home Act of 2018 (see Table 1 for an estimate of the direct spending effects of H.R. 5808)
- H.R. 5812, Creating Opportunities that Necessitate New and Enhanced Connections That Improve Opioid Navigation Strategies Act (CONNECTIONS) Act

Pay-As-You-Go considerations: The Statutory Pay-As-You-Go Act of 2010 establishes budget-reporting and enforcement procedures for legislation affecting direct spending or revenues. Twenty-two of the bills discussed in this document contain direct spending or revenues and are subject to pay-as-you-go procedures. Details about the amount of direct spending and revenues in those bills can be found in Table 1.

Increase in long-term direct spending and deficits: CBO estimates that enacting H.R. 4998, the Health Insurance for Former Foster Youth Act, would increase net direct spending by more than $2.5 billion and on-budget deficits by more than $5 billion in at least one of the four consecutive 10-year periods beginning in 2029. CBO estimates that none of the remaining 58 bills included in this estimate would increase net direct spending by more than $2.5 billion or on-budget deficits by more than $5 billion in any of the four consecutive 10-year periods beginning in 2029.

Mandates: One of the 59 bills included in this document, H.R. 5795, would impose both intergovernmental and private-sector mandates as defined in UMRA. CBO estimates that the costs of that bill's mandates on public and private entities would fall below UMRA's thresholds ($80 million and $160 million, respectively, for public- and private-sector entities in 2018, adjusted annually for inflation).

In addition, five bills would impose private-sector mandates as defined in UMRA. CBO estimates that the costs of the mandates in three of those bills (H.R. 5333, H.R. 5554, and H.R. 5811) would fall below the UMRA threshold. Because CBO does not know how federal agencies would implement new authority granted in the other two of those five bills, H.R. 5228 and 5687, CBO cannot determine whether the costs of their mandates would exceed the threshold.

For large entitlement grant programs, including Medicaid and CHIP, UMRA defines an increase in the stringency of conditions on states or localities as an intergovernmental mandate if the affected governments lack authority to offset those costs while continuing to provide required services. Because states possess significant flexibility to alter their responsibilities within Medicaid and CHIP, the requirements imposed by various bills in the markup on state administration of those programs would not constitute mandates as defined in UMRA.

## Mandates Affecting Public and Private Entities

H.R. 5795, the Overdose Prevention and Patient Safety Act, would impose intergovernmental and private-sector mandates by requiring entities that provide treatment for substance use disorders to notify patients of their privacy rights and also to notify patients in the event that the confidentiality of their records is breached. In certain circumstances, H.R. 5795 also would prohibit public and private entities from denying entry to treatment on the basis of information in patient health records. Those requirements would either supplant or narrowly expand responsibilities under existing law, and compliance with them would not impose significant additional costs. CBO estimates that the costs of the mandates would fall below the annual thresholds established in UMRA.

## Mandates Affecting Private Entities

Five bills included in this document would impose private-sector mandates:

*H.R. 5228, the Stop Counterfeit Drugs by Regulating and Enhancing Enforcement Now Act,* would require drug distributors to cease distributing any drug that the Secretary of HHS determines might present an imminent or substantial hazard to public health. CBO cannot determine what drugs could be subject to such an order nor can it determine how private entities would respond. Consequently, CBO cannot determine whether the aggregate cost of the mandate would exceed the annual threshold for private-sector mandates.

*H.R. 5333, the Over-the-Counter Monograph Safety, Innovation, and Reform Act of 2018,* would require developers and manufacturers of OTC drugs to pay certain fees to the FDA. CBO estimates that about $30 million would be collected each year, on average, for a total of $147 million over the 2019–2023 period. Those amounts would not exceed the annual threshold for private-sector mandates in any year during that period.

*H.R. 5554, the Animal Drug and Animal Generic Drug User Fee Amendments of 2018*, would require developers and manufacturers of brand-name and generic veterinary drugs to pay application, product, establishment, and sponsor fees to the FDA. CBO estimates that about $51 million would be collected annually, on average, for a total of $257 million over the 2019–2023 period. Those amounts would not exceed the annual threshold for private-sector mandates in any year during that period.

*H.R. 5687, the Securing Opioids and Unused Narcotics with Deliberate Disposal and Packaging Act of 2018,* would permit the Secretary of HHS to require drug developers and manufacturers to implement new packaging and disposal technology for certain drugs. Based on information from the agency, CBO expects that the Secretary would use the new regulatory authority provided in the bill; however, it is uncertain how or when those requirements would be implemented. Consequently, CBO cannot determine whether the aggregate cost of the mandate would exceed the annual threshold for private entities.

*H.R. 5811, a bill to amend the Federal Food, Drug, and Cosmetic Act with respect to postapproval study requirements for certain controlled substances, and for other purposes,* would expand an existing mandate that requires drug developers to conduct postapproval studies or clinical trials for certain drugs. Under current law, in certain instances, the FDA can require studies or clinical trials after a drug has been approved. H.R. 5811 would permit the FDA to use that authority if the reduction in a drug's effectiveness meant that its benefits no longer outweighed its costs. CBO estimates that the incremental cost of the mandate would fall below the annual threshold established in UMRA because of the small number of drugs affected and the narrow expansion of the authority that exists under current law.

None of the remaining 53 bills included in this document would impose an intergovernmental or private-sector mandate.

Previous CBO estimate: On June 6, 2018, CBO issued an estimate for seven opioid-related bills ordered reported by the House Committee on Ways and Means on May 16, 2018. Two of those bills contain provisions that are identical or similar to the legislation ordered reported by the Committee on Energy and Commerce, and for those provisions, CBO's estimates are the same.

In particular, five bills listed in this estimate contain provisions that are identical or similar to those in several sections of H.R. 5773, the Preventing Addiction for Susceptible Seniors Act of 2018:

- H.R. 5675, which would require prescription drug plans to implement drug management programs, is identical to section 2 of H.R. 5773.
- H.R. 4841, regarding electronic prior authorization for prescriptions under Medicare's Part D, is similar to section 3 of H.R. 5773.

- H.R. 5715, which would mandate the creation of a new Internet portal to allow various stakeholders to exchange information, is identical to section 4 of H.R. 5773.
- H.R. 5684, which would expand medication therapy management, is the same as section 5 of H.R. 5773.
- H.R. 5716, regarding prescriber notification, is identical to section 6 of H.R. 5773.

In addition, in this estimate, a provision related to Medicare beneficiary education in H.R. 5686, the Medicare Clear Health Options in Care for Enrollees Act of 2018, is the same as a provision in section 2 of H.R. 5775, the Providing Reliable Options for Patients and Educational Resources Act of 2018, in CBO's estimate for the Committee on Ways and Means.

Estimate prepared by: Federal Costs: Rebecca Yip (Centers for Disease Control and Prevention), Mark Grabowicz (Drug Enforcement Agency), Julia Christensen, Ellen Werble (Food and Drug Administration), Emily King, Andrea Noda, Lisa Ramirez-Branum, Robert Stewart (Medicaid and Children's Health Insurance Program), Philippa Haven, Lara Robillard, Colin Yee, Rebecca Yip (Medicare), Philippa Haven (National Institutes of Health), Alice Burns, Andrea Noda (Office of the Secretary of the Department of Health and Human Services), Philippa Haven, Lori Housman, Emily King (Substance Abuse and Mental Health Services Administration, Health Resources and Services Administration); Federal Revenues: Jacob Fabian, Peter Huether, and Cecilia Pastrone; Fact Checking: Zachary Byrum and Kate Kelly; Mandates: Andrew Laughlin.

Estimate reviewed by: Tom Bradley, Chief, Health Systems and Medicare Cost Estimates Unit; Chad M. Chirico, Chief, Low-Income Health Programs and Prescription Drugs Cost Estimates Unit; Sarah Masi, Special Assistant for Health; Susan Willie, Chief, Mandates Unit; Leo Lex, Deputy Assistant Director for Budget Analysis; Theresa A. Gullo, Assistant Director for Budget Analysis.

## Federal Mandates Statement

The Committee adopts as its own the estimate of Federal mandates prepared by the Director of the Congressional Budget Office pursuant to section 423 of the Unfunded Mandates Reform Act.

## Statement of General Performance Goals and Objectives

Pursuant to clause 3(c)(4) of rule XIII, the general performance goal or objective of this legislation is work with eligible entities, including Quality Improvement Organizations, to instruct Centers for Medicare and Medicaid Services (CMS) to add a review of current opioid prescriptions and, as appropriate, a screening for opioid use disorder as part of the Welcome to Medicare initial examination.

## Duplication of Federal Programs

Pursuant to clause 3(c)(5) of rule XIII, no provision of H.R. 5798 is known to be duplicative of another Federal program, including any program that was included in a report to Congress pursuant to section 21 of Public Law 111–139 or the most recent Catalog of Federal Domestic Assistance.

## Committee Cost Estimate

Pursuant to clause 3(d)(1) of rule XIII, the Committee adopts as its own the cost estimate prepared by the Director of the Congressional Budget Office pursuant to section 402 of the Congressional Budget Act of 1974.

## Earmark, Limited Tax Benefits, and Limited Tariff Benefits

Pursuant to clause 9(e), 9(f), and 9(g) of rule XXI, the Committee finds that H.R. 5798 contains no earmarks, limited tax benefits, or limited tariff benefits.

## Disclosure of Directed Rule Makings

Pursuant to section 3(i) of H. Res. 5, the Committee finds that H.R. 3331 contains no directed rule makings.

## Advisory Committee Statement

No advisory committees within the meaning of section 5(b) of the Federal Advisory Committee Act were created by this legislation.

## Applicability to Legislative Branch

The Committee finds that the legislation does not relate to the terms and conditions of employment or access to public services or accommodations within the meaning of section 102(b)(3) of the Congressional Accountability Act.

## Section-by-Section Analysis of the Legislation

### Section 1. Short Title

The section provides that the Act may be cited as the "Opioid Screening and Chronic Management Alternatives for Seniors Act."

**Section 2. Requiring a Review of Current Opioid Prescriptions for Chronic Pain and Screening for Opioid Use Disorder to Be Included in the Welcome to Medicare Initial Preventive Physical Examination**

Section 2 provides that an Initial Preventive Physical Examination shall include a review of current opioid prescriptions and screenings for opioid use disorder.

## CHANGES IN EXISTING LAW MADE BY THE BILL, AS REPORTED

In compliance with clause 3(e) of rule XIII of the Rules of the House of Representatives, changes in existing law made by the bill, as reported, are shown as follows (new matter is printed in italic and existing law in which no change is proposed is shown in roman):

**Social Security Act**

Title XVIII—Health Insurance For The Aged And Disabled Part E—Miscellaneous Provisions Definitions Of Services, Institutions, Etc.

SEC. 1861. For purposes of this title—

***Spell of Illness***

(a) The term "spell of illness" with respect to any individual means a period of consecutive days—

(1) beginning with the first day (not included in a previous spell of illness) (A) on which such individual is furnished inpatient hospital services, inpatient critical access hospital services or extended care services, and (B) which occurs in a month for which he is entitled to benefits under part A, and

(2) ending with the close of the first period of 60 consecutive days thereafter on each of which he is neither an inpatient of a hospital or critical access hospital nor an inpatient of a facility described in section 1819(a)(1) or subsection (y)(1).

***Inpatient Hospital Services***

(b) The term "inpatient hospital services" means the following items and services furnished to an inpatient of a hospital and (except as provided in paragraph (3)) by the hospital—

(1) bed and board;

(2) such nursing services and other related services, such use of hospital facilities, and such medical social services as are ordinarily furnished by the hospital for the care and treatment of inpatients, and such drugs, biologicals, supplies, appliances, and equipment, for use in the hospital, as are ordinarily furnished by such hospital for the care and treatment of inpatients; and

(3) such other diagnostic or therapeutic items or services, furnished by the hospital or by others under arrangements with them made by the hospital, as are ordinarily furnished to inpatients either by such hospital or by others under such arrangements;

excluding, however—

(4) medical or surgical services provided by a physician, resident, or intern, services described by subsection (s)(2)(K), certified nurse-midwife services, qualified psychologist services, and services of a certified registered nurse anesthetist; and

(5) the services of a private-duty nurse or other private-duty attendant.

Paragraph (4) shall not apply to services provided in a hospital by—

(6) an intern or a resident-in-training under a teaching program approved by the Council on Medical Education of the American Medical Association or, in the case of an osteopathic hospital, approved by the Committee on Hospitals of the Bureau of Professional Education of the American Osteopathic Association, or, in the case of services in a hospital or osteopathic hospital by an intern or resident-in-training in the field of dentistry, approved by the Council on Dental Education of the American

Dental Association, or in the case of services in a hospital or osteopathic hospital by an intern or resident-in-training in the field of podiatry, approved by the Council on Podiatric Medical Education of the American Podiatric Medical Association; or

(7) a physician where the hospital has a teaching program approved as specified in paragraph (6), if (A) the hospital elects to receive any payment due under this title for reasonable costs of such services, and (B) all physicians in such hospital agree not to bill charges for professional services rendered in such hospital to individuals covered under the insurance program established by this title.

***Inpatient Psychiatric Hospital Services***

(c) The term "inpatient psychiatric hospital services" means inpatient hospital services furnished to an inpatient of a psychiatric hospital.

***Supplier***

(d) The term "supplier" means, unless the context otherwise requires, a physician or other practitioner, a facility, or other entity (other than a provider of services) that furnishes items or services under this title.

***Hospital***

(e) The term "hospital" (except for purposes of sections 1814(d), 1814(f), and 1835(b), subsection (a)(2) of this section, paragraph (7) of this subsection, and subsection (i) of this section) means an institution which—

(1) is primarily engaged in providing, by or under the supervision of physicians, to inpatients (A) diagnostic services and therapeutic services for medical diagnosis, treatment, and care of injured, disabled, or sick persons, or (B) rehabilitation services for the rehabilitation of injured, disabled, or sick persons;

(2) maintains clinical records on all patients;

(3) has bylaws in effect with respect to its staff of physicians;

(4) has a requirement that every patient with respect to whom payment may be made under this title must be under the care of a physician, except that a patient receiving qualified psychologist services (as defined in

subsection (ii)) may be under the care of a clinical psychologist with respect to such services to the extent permitted under State law;

(5) provides 24-hour nursing service rendered or supervised by a registered professional nurse, and has a licensed practical nurse or registered professional nurse on duty at all times; except that until January 1, 1979, the Secretary is authorized to waive the requirement of this paragraph for any one-year period with respect to any institution, insofar as such requirement relates to the provision of twenty-four-hour nursing service rendered or supervised by a registered professional nurse (except that in any event a registered professional nurse must be present on the premises to render or supervise the nursing service provided, during at least the regular daytime shift), where immediately preceding such one-year period he finds that—

(A) such institution is located in a rural area and the supply of hospital services in such area is not sufficient to meet the needs of individuals residing therein,

(B) the failure of such institution to qualify as a hospital would seriously reduce the availability of such services to such individuals, and

(C) such institution has made and continues to make a good faith effort to comply with this paragraph, but such compliance is impeded by the lack of qualified nursing personnel in such area;

(6)(A) has in effect a hospital utilization review plan which meets the requirements of subsection (k) and (B) has in place a discharge planning process that meets the requirements of subsection (ee);

(7) in the case of an institution in any State in which State or applicable local law provides for the licensing of hospitals,

(A) is licensed pursuant to such law or (B) is approved, by the agency of such State or locality responsible for licensing hospitals, as meeting the standards established for such licensing;

(8) has in effect an overall plan and budget that meets the requirements of subsection (z); and

(9) meets such other requirements as the Secretary finds necessary in the interest of the health and safety of individuals who are furnished services in the institution.

For purposes of subsection (a)(2), such term includes any institution which meets the requirements of paragraph (1) of this subsection. For purposes of sections 1814(d) and 1835(b) (including determination of whether an individual received inpatient hospital services or diagnostic services for purposes of such sections), section 1814(f)(2), and subsection (i) of this section, such term includes any institution which (i) meets the requirements of paragraphs (5) and (7) of this subsection, (ii) is not primarily engaged in providing the services described in section 1861(j)(1)(A) and (iii) is primarily engaged in providing, by or under the supervision of individuals referred to in paragraph (1) of section 1861(r), to inpatients diagnostic services and therapeutic services for medical diagnosis, treatment, and care of injured, disabled, or sick persons, or rehabilitation services for the rehabilitation of injured, disabled, or sick persons. For purposes of section 1814(f)(1), such term includes an institution which (i) is a hospital for purposes of sections 1814(d), 1814(f)(2), and 1835(b) and (ii) is accredited by a national accreditation body recognized by the Secretary under section 1865(a), or is accredited by or approved by a program of the country in which such institution is located if the Secretary finds the accreditation or comparable approval standards of such program to be essentially equivalent to those of such a national accreditation body. Notwith-standing the preceding provisions of this subsection, such term shall not, except for purposes of subsection (a)(2), include any institution which is primarily for the care and treatment of mental diseases unless it is a psychiatric hospital (as defined in subsection (f)). The term "hospital" also includes a religious nonmedical health care institution (as defined in subsection (ss)(1)), but only with respect to items and services ordinarily furnished by such institution to inpatients, and payment may be made with respect to services provided by or in such an institution only to such extent and under such conditions, limitations, and requirements (in addition to or in lieu of the conditions, limitations, and requirements otherwise applicable) as may be provided in regulations consistent with section 1821. For provisions deeming certain requirements of this subsection to be met in the case of accredited institutions, see section 1865. The term "hospital" also includes a facility of fifty beds or less which is located in an area determined by the Secretary to meet the definition relating to a rural area described in subparagraph (A) of paragraph (5) of this subsection and which meets the other requirements of this subsection, except that—

(A) with respect to the requirements for nursing services applicable after December 31, 1978, such requirements shall provide for temporary waiver of the requirements, for such period as the Secretary deems appropriate, where (i) the facility's failure to fully comply with the requirements is attributable to a temporary shortage of qualified nursing personnel in the area in which the facility is located, (ii) a registered professional nurse is present on the premises to render or supervise the nursing service provided during at least the regular daytime shift, and (iii) the Secretary determines that the employment of such nursing personnel as are available to the facility during such temporary period will not adversely affect the health and safety of patients;

(B) with respect to the health and safety requirements promulgated under paragraph (9), such requirements shall be applied by the Secretary to a facility herein defined in such manner as to assure that personnel requirements take into account the availability of technical personnel and the educational opportunities for technical personnel in the area in which such facility is located, and the scope of services rendered by such facility; and the Secretary, by regulations, shall provide for the continued participation of such a facility where such personnel requirements are not fully met, for such period as the Secretary determines that (i) the facility is making good faith efforts to fully comply with the personnel requirements, (ii) the employment by the facility of such personnel as are available to the facility will not adversely affect the health and safety of patients, and (iii) if the Secretary has determined that because of the facility's waiver under this subparagraph the facility should limit its scope of services in order not to adversely affect the health and safety of the facility's patients, the facility is so limiting the scope of services it provides; and

(C) with respect to the fire and safety requirements promulgated under paragraph (9), the Secretary (i) may waive, for such period as he deems appropriate, specific provisions of such requirements which if rigidly applied would result in unreasonable hardship for such a facility and which, if not applied, would not jeopardize the health and safety of patients, and (ii) may accept a facility's compliance with all applicable State codes relating to fire and safety in lieu of compliance with the fire and safety requirements promulgated under paragraph (9), if he determines that such State has in effect fire and safety codes, imposed by State law, which adequately protect patients.

The term "hospital" does not include, unless the context otherwise requires, a critical access hospital (as defined in section 1861(mm)(1)).

***Psychiatric Hospital***

(f) The term "psychiatric hospital" means an institution which—

(1) is primarily engaged in providing, by or under the supervision of a physician, psychiatric services for the diagnosis and treatment of mentally ill persons;

(2) satisfies the requirements of paragraphs (3) through (9) of subsection (e);

(3) maintains clinical records on all patients and maintains such records as the Secretary finds to be necessary to determine the degree and intensity of the treatment provided to individuals entitled to hospital insurance benefits under part A; and

(4) meets such staffing requirements as the Secretary finds necessary for the institution to carry out an active program of treatment for individuals who are furnished services in the institution.

In the case of an institution which satisfies paragraphs (1) and (2) of the preceding sentence and which contains a distinct part which also satisfies paragraphs (3) and (4) of such sentence, such distinct part shall be considered to be a "psychiatric hospital."

***Outpatient Occupational Therapy Services***

(g) The term "outpatient occupational therapy services" has the meaning given the term "outpatient physical therapy services" in subsection (p), except that "occupational" shall be substituted for "physical" each place it appears therein.

***Extended Care Services***

(h) The term "extended care services" means the following items and services furnished to an inpatient of a skilled nursing facility and (except as provided in paragraphs (3), (6) and (7)) by such skilled nursing facility—

(1) nursing care provided by or under the supervision of a registered professional nurse;

(2) bed and board in connection with the furnishing of such nursing care;

(3) physical or occupational therapy or speech-language pathology services furnished by the skilled nursing facility or by others under arrangements with them made by the facility;

(4) medical social services;

(5) such drugs, biologicals, supplies, appliances, and equipment, furnished for use in the skilled nursing facility, as are ordinarily furnished by such facility for the care and treatment of inpatients;

(6) medical services provided by an intern or resident-in-training of a hospital with which the facility has in effect a transfer agreement (meeting the requirements of subsection (l)), under a teaching program of such hospital approved as provided in the last sentence of subsection (b), and other diagnostic or therapeutic services provided by a hospital with which the facility has such an agreement in effect; and

(7) such other services necessary to the health of the patients as are generally provided by skilled nursing facilities, or by others under arrangements with them made by the facility; excluding, however, any item or service if it would not be included under subsection (b) if furnished to an inpatient of a hospital.

***Post-Hospital Extended Care Services***

(i) The term "post-hospital extended care services" means extended care services furnished an individual after transfer from a hospital in which he was an inpatient for not less than 3 consecutive days before his discharge from the hospital in connection with such transfer. For purposes of the preceding sentence, items and services shall be deemed to have been furnished to an individual after transfer from a hospital, and he shall be deemed to have been an inpatient in the hospital immediately before transfer therefrom, if he is admitted to the skilled nursing facility (A) within 30 days after discharge from such hospital, or (B) within such time as it would be medically appropriate to begin an active course of treatment, in the case of an individual whose condition is such that skilled nursing facility care would not be medically appropriate within 30 days after discharge from a hospital; and an individual shall be deemed not to have been discharged from a skilled nursing facility if, within 30 days after discharge therefrom, he is admitted to such facility or any other skilled nursing facility.

***Skilled Nursing Facility***

(j) The term "skilled nursing facility" has the meaning given such term in section 1819(a).

***Utilization Review***

(k) A utilization review plan of a hospital or skilled nursing facility shall be considered sufficient if it is applicable to services furnished by the institution to individuals entitled to insurance benefits under this title and if it provides—

(1) for the review, on a sample or other basis, of admissions to the institution, the duration of stays therein, and the professional services (including drugs and biologicals) furnished, (A) with respect to the medical necessity of the services, and (B) for the purpose of promoting the most efficient use of available health facilities and services;

(2) for such review to be made by either (A) a staff committee of the institution composed of two or more physicians (of which at least two must be physicians described in subsection (r)(1) of this section), with or without participation of other professional personnel, or (B) a group outside the institution which is similarly composed and (i) which is established by the local medical society and some or all of the hospitals and skilled nursing facilities in the locality, or (ii) if (and for as long as) there has not been established such a group which serves such institution,

which is established in such other manner as may be approved by the Secretary;

(3) for such review, in each case of inpatient hospital services or extended care services furnished to such an individual during a continuous period of extended duration, as of such days of such period (which may differ for different classes of cases) as may be specified in regulations, with such review to be made as promptly as possible, after each day so specified, and in no event later than one week following such day; and

(4) for prompt notification to the institution, the individual, and his attending physician of any finding (made after opportunity for consultation to such attending physician) by the physician members of such committee or group that any further stay in the institution is not medically necessary.

The review committee must be composed as provided in clause (B) of paragraph (2) rather than as provided in clause (A) of such paragraph in the case of any hospital or skilled nursing facility where, because of the small size of the institution, or (in the case of a skilled nursing facility) because of lack of an organized medical staff, or for such other reason or reasons as may be included in regulations, it is impracticable for the institution to have a properly functioning staff committee for the purposes of this subsection. If the Secretary determines that the utilization review procedures established pursuant to title XIX are superior in their effectiveness to the procedures required under this section, he may, to the extent that he deems it appropriate, require for purposes of this title that the procedures established pursuant to title XIX be utilized instead of the procedures required by this section.

### *Agreements for Transfer between Skilled Nursing Facilities and Hospitals*

(L) A hospital and a skilled nursing facility shall be considered to have a transfer agreement in effect if, by reason of a written agreement between them or (in case the two institutions are under common control) by reason of a written undertaking by the person or body which controls them, there is reasonable assurance that—

(1) transfer of patients will be effected between the hospital and the skilled nursing facility whenever such transfer is medically appropriate as determined by the attending physician; and

(2) there will be interchange of medical and other information necessary or useful in the care and treatment of individuals transferred between the institutions, or in determining whether such individuals can be adequately cared for otherwise than in either of such institutions.

Any skilled nursing facility which does not have such an agreement in effect, but which is found by a State agency (of the State in which such facility is situated) with which an agreement under section 1864 is in effect (or, in the case of a State in which no such agency has an agreement under section 1864, by the Secretary) to have attempted in good faith to enter into such an agreement with a hospital sufficiently close to the facility to make feasible the transfer between them of patients and the information referred to in paragraph (2), shall be considered to have such an agreement in effect if and for so long as such agency (or the Secretary, as the case may be) finds that to do so is in the public interest and essential to assuring extended care services for persons in the community who are eligible for payments with respect to such services under this title.

### *Home Health Services*

(m) The term "home health services" means the following items and services furnished to an individual, who is under the care of a physician, by a home health agency or by others under arrangements with them made by such agency, under a plan (for furnishing such items and services to such individual) established and periodically reviewed by a physician, which items and services are, except as provided in paragraph (7), provided on a visiting basis in a place of residence used as such individual's home—

(1) part-time or intermittent nursing care provided by or under the supervision of a registered professional nurse;

(2) physical or occupational therapy or speech-language pathology services;

(3) medical social services under the direction of a physician;

(4) to the extent permitted in regulations, part-time or intermittent services of a home health aide who has successfully completed a training program approved by the Secretary;

(5) medical supplies (including catheters, catheter supplies, ostomy bags, and supplies related to ostomy care, and a covered osteoporosis drug (as defined in subsection (kk)), but excluding other drugs and biologicals) and durable medical equipment and applicable disposable devices (as defined in section 1834(s)(2)) while under such a plan;

(6) in the case of a home health agency which is affiliated or under common control with a hospital, medical services provided by an intern or resident-in-training of such hospital, under a teaching program of such hospital approved as provided in the last sentence of subsection (b); and

(7) any of the foregoing items and services which are provided on an outpatient basis, under arrangements made by the home health agency, at a hospital or skilled nursing facility, or at a rehabilitation center which meets such standards as may be prescribed in regulations, and—

(A) the furnishing of which involves the use of equipment of such a nature that the items and services cannot readily be made available to the individual in such place of residence, or

(B) which are furnished at such facility while he is there to receive any such item or service described in clause (A), but not including transportation of the individual in connection with any such item or service; excluding, however, any item or service if it would not be included under subsection (b) if furnished to an inpatient of a hospital and home infusion therapy (as defined in subsection (iii)(i)). For purposes of paragraphs (1) and (4), the term "part-time or intermittent services" means skilled nursing and home health aide services furnished any number of days per week as long as they are furnished (combined) less than 8 hours each day and 28 or fewer hours each week (or, subject to review on a case-by-case basis as to the need for care, less than 8 hours each day and 35 or fewer hours per week). For purposes of sections 1814(a)(2)(C) and 1835(a)(2)(A), "intermittent" means skilled nursing care that is either provided or needed on fewer than 7 days each week, or less than 8 hours of each day for periods of 21 days or less (with extensions in exceptional circumstances when the need for additional care is finite and predictable).

### Durable Medical Equipment

(n) The term "durable medical equipment" includes iron lungs, oxygen tents, hospital beds, and wheelchairs (which may include a power-operated vehicle that may be appropriately used as a wheel-chair, but only where the use of such a vehicle is determined to be necessary on the basis of the individual's medical and physical condition and the vehicle meets such safety requirements as the Secretary may prescribe) used in the patient's home (including an institution used as his home other than an institution that meets the requirements of subsection (e)(1) of this section or section 1819(a)(1)), whether furnished on a rental basis or purchased, and includes blood-testing strips and blood glucose monitors for individuals with diabetes without regard to whether the individual has Type I or Type II diabetes or to the individual's use of insulin (as determined under standards established by the Secretary in consultation with the appropriate organizations) and eye tracking and gaze interaction accessories for speech generating devices furnished to individuals with a demonstrated medical need for such accessories; except that such term does not include such equipment furnished by a supplier who has used, for the demonstration and use of specific equipment, an individual who has not met such minimum training standards as the Secretary may establish with respect to the demonstration and use of such specific equipment. With respect to a seat-lift chair, such term includes only the seat-lift mechanism and does not include the chair.

### Home Health Agency

(o) The term "home health agency" means a public agency or private organization, or a subdivision of such an agency or organization, which—

(1) is primarily engaged in providing skilled nursing services and other therapeutic services;

(2) has policies, established by a group of professional personnel (associated with the agency or organization), including one or more

physicians and one or more registered professional nurses, to govern the services (referred to in paragraph (1)) which it provides, and provides for supervision of such services by a physician or registered professional nurse;

(3) maintains clinical records on all patients;

(4) in the case of an agency or organization in any State in which State or applicable local law provides for the licensing of agencies or organizations of this nature, (A) is licensed pursuant to such law, or (B) is approved, by the agency of such State or locality responsible for licensing agencies or organizations of this nature, as meeting the standards established for such licensing;

(5) has in effect an overall plan and budget that meets the requirements of subsection (z);

(6) meets the conditions of participation specified in section 1891(a) and such other conditions of participation as the Secretary may find necessary in the interest of the health and safety of individuals who are furnished services by such agency or organization;

(7) provides the Secretary with a surety bond—

(A) in a form specified by the Secretary and in an amount that is not less than the minimum of $50,000; and

(B) that the Secretary determines is commensurate with the volume of payments to the home health agency; and

(8) meets such additional requirements (including conditions relating to bonding or establishing of escrow accounts as the Secretary finds necessary for the financial security of the program) as the Secretary finds necessary for the effective and efficient operation of the program; except that for purposes of part A such term shall not include any agency or organization which is primarily for the care and treatment of mental diseases. The Secretary may waive the requirement of a surety bond under paragraph (7) in the case of an agency or organization that provides a comparable surety bond under State law.

***Outpatient Physical Therapy Services***

(p) The term "outpatient physical therapy services" means physical therapy services furnished by a provider of services, a clinic, rehabilitation agency, or a public health agency, or by others under an arrangement with, and under the supervision of, such provider, clinic, rehabilitation agency, or public health agency to an individual as an outpatient—

(1) who is under the care of a physician (as defined in paragraph (1), (3), or (4) of section 1861(r)), and

(2) with respect to whom a plan prescribing the type, amount, and duration of physical therapy services that are to be furnished such individual has been established by a physician (as so defined) or by a qualified physical therapist and is periodically reviewed by a physician (as so defined);

excluding, however—

(3) any item or service if it would not be included under subsection (b) if furnished to an inpatient of a hospital; and

(4) any such service—

(A) if furnished by a clinic or rehabilitation agency, or by others under arrangements with such clinic or agency, unless such clinic or rehabilitation agency—

(i) provides an adequate program of physical therapy services for outpatients and has the facilities and personnel required for such program or required for the supervision of such a program, in accordance with such requirements as the Secretary may specify,

(ii) has policies, established by a group of professional personnel, including one or more physicians (associated with the clinic or rehabilitation agency) and one or more qualified physical therapists, to govern the services (referred to in clause (i)) it provides,

(iii) maintains clinical records on all patients,

(iv) if such clinic or agency is situated in a State in which State or applicable local law provides for the licensing of institutions of this nature, (I) is licensed pursuant to such law, or (II) is approved by the agency of such State or locality responsible for licensing institutions of this nature, as meeting the standards established for such licensing; and

(v) meets such other conditions relating to the health and safety of individuals who are furnished services by such clinic or agency on an outpatient basis, as the Secretary may find necessary, and provides the Secretary on a continuing basis with a surety bond in a form specified by the Secretary and in an amount that is not less than $50,000, or

(B) if furnished by a public health agency, unless such agency meets such other conditions relating to health and safety of individuals who are furnished services by such agency on an outpatient basis, as the Secretary may find necessary.

The term "outpatient physical therapy services" also includes physical therapy services furnished an individual by a physical therapist (in his office or in such individual's home) who meets licensing and other standards prescribed by the Secretary in regulations, otherwise than under an arrangement with and under the supervision of a provider of services, clinic, rehabilitation agency, or public health agency, if the furnishing of such services meets such conditions relating to health and safety as the Secretary may find necessary. In addition, such term includes physical therapy services which meet the requirements of the first sentence of this subsection except that they are furnished to an individual as an inpatient of a hospital or extended care facility. Nothing in this subsection shall be construed as requiring, with respect to outpatients who are not entitled to benefits under this title, a physical therapist to provide outpatient physical therapy services only to outpatients who are under the care of a physician or pursuant to a plan of care established by a physician. The Secretary may waive the requirement of a surety bond under paragraph (4)(A)(v) in the case of a clinic or agency that provides a comparable surety bond under State law.

***Physicians' Services***

(q) The term "physicians' services" means professional services performed by physicians, including surgery, consultation, and home, office, and institutional calls (but not including services described in subsection (b)(6)).

***Physician***

(r) The term "physician," when used in connection with the performance of any function or action, means (1) a doctor of medicine or osteopathy legally authorized to practice medicine and surgery by the State in which he performs such function or action (including a physician within the meaning of section 1101(a)(7)), (2) a doctor of dental surgery or of dental medicine who is legally authorized to practice dentistry by the State in which he performs such function and who is acting within the scope of his license when he performs such functions, (3) a doctor of podiatric medicine for the purposes of subsections (k), (m), (p)(1), and (s) of this section and sections 1814(a), 1832(a)(2)(F)(ii), and 1835 but only with respect to functions which he is legally authorized to perform as such by the State in which he performs them, (4) a doctor of optometry, but only for purposes of subsection (p)(1) and with respect to the provision of items or services described in subsection (s) which he is legally authorized to perform as a doctor of optometry by the State in which he performs them, or (5) a chiropractor who is licensed as such by the State (or in a State which does not license chiropractors as such, is legally authorized to perform the services of a chiropractor in the jurisdiction in which he performs such services), and who meets uniform minimum standards promulgated by the Secretary, but only for the purpose of sections 1861(s)(1) and 1861(s)(2)(A) and only with respect to treatment by means of manual manipulation of the spine (to correct a subluxation) which he is legally authorized to perform by the State or jurisdiction in which such treatment is provided. For the purposes of section 1862(a)(4) and subject to the limitations and conditions provided in the previous sentence, such term includes a doctor of one of the arts, specified in such previous sentence, legally authorized to practice such art in the country in which the inpatient hospital services (referred to in such section 1862(a)(4)) are furnished.

***Medical and Other Health Services***

(s) The term "medical and other health services" means any of the following items or services:

(1) physicians' services;

(2) (A) services and supplies (including drugs and biologicals which are not usually self-administered by the patient) furnished as an incident to a physician's professional service, of kinds which are commonly furnished in physicians' offices and are commonly either rendered without charge or included in the physicians' bills (or would have been so included but for the application of section 1847B);

(B) hospital services (including drugs and biologicals which are not usually self-administered by the patient) incident to physicians' services rendered to outpatients and partial hospitalization services incident to such services;

(C) diagnostic services which are—

(i) furnished to an individual as an outpatient by a hospital or by others under arrangements with them made by a hospital, and

(ii) ordinarily furnished by such hospital (or by others under such arrangements) to its outpatients for the purpose of diagnostic study;

(D) outpatient physical therapy services, outpatient speech-language pathology services, and outpatient occupational therapy services;

(E) rural health clinic services and Federally qualified health center services;

(F) home dialysis supplies and equipment, self-care home dialysis support services, and institutional dialysis services and supplies, and, for items and services furnished on or after January 1, 2011, renal dialysis services (as defined in section 1881(b)(14)(B)), including such renal dialysis services furnished on or after January 1, 2017, by a renal dialysis facility or provider of services paid under section 1881(b)(14) to an individual with acute kidney injury (as defined in section 1834(r)(2));

(G) antigens (subject to quantity limitations prescribed in regulations by the Secretary) prepared by a physician, as defined in section 1861(r)(1), for a particular patient, including antigens so prepared which are forwarded to another qualified person (including a rural health clinic) for administration to such patient, from time to time, by or under the supervision of another such physician;

(H) (i) services furnished pursuant to a contract under section 1876 to a member of an eligible organization by a physician assistant or by a nurse practitioner (as defined in subsection (aa)(5)) and such services and supplies furnished as an incident to his service to such a member as would otherwise be covered under this part if furnished by a physician or as an incident to a physician's service; and

(ii) services furnished pursuant to a risk-sharing contract under section 1876(g) to a member of an eligible organization by a clinical psychologist (as defined by the Secretary) or by a clinical social worker (as defined in subsection (hh)(2)), and such services and supplies furnished as an incident to such clinical psychologist's services or clinical social worker's services to such a member as would otherwise be covered under this part if furnished by a physician or as an incident to a physician's service;

(I) blood clotting factors, for hemophilia patients competent to use such factors to control bleeding without medical or other supervision, and items related to the administration of such factors, subject to utilization controls deemed necessary by the Secretary for the efficient use of such factors;

(J) prescription drugs used in immunosuppressive therapy furnished, to an individual who receives an organ transplant for which payment is made under this title;

(K) (i) services which would be physicians' services and services described in subsections (ww)(1) and (hhh) if furnished by a physician (as defined in subsection (r)(1)) and which are performed by a physician assistant (as defined in subsection (aa)(5)) under the supervision of a physician (as so defined) and which the physician assistant is legally authorized to perform by the State in which the services are performed, and such services and supplies furnished as incident to such services as would be covered under subparagraph (A) if furnished incident to a physician's professional service, but only if no facility or other provider charges or is paid any amounts with respect to the furnishing of such services,

(ii) services which would be physicians' services and services described in subsections (ww)(1) and (hhh) if furnished by a physician (as defined in subsection (r)(1)) and which are performed by a nurse practitioner or clinical nurse specialist (as defined in subsection (aa)(5)) working in collaboration (as defined in subsection (aa)(6)) with a physician (as defined in sub-section (r)(1)) which the nurse practitioner or clinical nurse specialist is legally authorized to perform by the State in which the services are performed, and such services and supplies furnished as an incident to such services as would be covered under subparagraph (A) if furnished incident to a physician's professional service, but only if no facility or other provider charges or is paid any amounts with respect to the furnishing of such services;

(L) certified nurse-midwife services;

(M) qualified psychologist services;

(N) clinical social worker services (as defined in subsection (hh)(2));

(O) erythropoietin for dialysis patients competent to use such drug without medical or other supervision with respect to the administration of such drug, subject to methods and standards established by the Secretary by regulation for the safe and effective use of such drug, and items related to the administration of such drug;

(P) prostate cancer screening tests (as defined in subsection (oo));

(Q) an oral drug (which is approved by the Federal Food and Drug Administration) prescribed for use as an anticancer chemotherapeutic agent for a given indication, and containing an active ingredient (or ingredients), which is the same indication and active ingredient (or ingredients) as a drug which the carrier determines would be covered pursuant to subparagraph

(A) or (B) if the drug could not be self-administered;

(R) colorectal cancer screening tests (as defined in subsection (pp));

(S) diabetes outpatient self-management training services (as defined in subsection (qq));

(T) an oral drug (which is approved by the Federal Food and Drug Administration) prescribed for use as an acute anti-emetic used as part of an anticancer chemotherapeutic regimen if the drug is administered by a physician (or as prescribed by a physician)—

(i) for use immediately before, at, or within 48 hours after the time of the administration of the anticancer chemotherapeutic agent; and

(ii) as a full replacement for the anti-emetic therapy which would otherwise be administered intravenously;

(U) screening for glaucoma (as defined in subsection (uu)) for individuals determined to be at high risk for glaucoma, individuals with a family history of glaucoma and individuals with diabetes;

(V) medical nutrition therapy services (as defined in subsection (vv)(1)) in the case of a beneficiary with diabetes or a renal disease who—

(i) has not received diabetes outpatient self-management training services within a time period determined by the Secretary;

(ii) is not receiving maintenance dialysis for which payment is made under section 1881; and

(iii) meets such other criteria determined by the Secretary after consideration of protocols established by dietitian or nutrition professional organizations;

(W) an initial preventive physical examination (as defined in subsection (ww));

(X) cardiovascular screening blood tests (as defined in subsection (xx)(1));

(Y) diabetes screening tests (as defined in subsection (yy));

(Z) intravenous immune globulin for the treatment of primary immune deficiency diseases in the home (as defined in subsection (zz));

(AA) ultrasound screening for abdominal aortic aneurysm (as defined in subsection (bbb)) for an individual—

(i) who receives a referral for such an ultrasound screening as a result of an initial preventive physical examination (as defined in section 1861(ww)(1));

(ii) who has not been previously furnished such an ultrasound screening under this title; and

(iii) who—

(I) has a family history of abdominal aortic aneurysm; or

(II) manifests risk factors included in a beneficiary category recommended for screening by the United States Preventive Services Task Force regarding abdominal aortic aneurysms;

(BB) additional preventive services (described in subsection (ddd)(1));

(CC) items and services furnished under a cardiac rehabilitation program (as defined in subsection (eee)(1)) or under a pulmonary rehabilitation program (as defined in subsection (fff)(1));

(DD) items and services furnished under an intensive cardiac rehabilitation program (as defined in subsection (eee)(4));

(EE) kidney disease education services (as defined in subsection (ggg));

(FF) personalized prevention plan services (as defined in subsection (hhh)); and

(GG) home infusion therapy (as defined in subsection (iii)(1));

(3) diagnostic X-ray tests (including tests under the supervision of a physician, furnished in a place of residence used as the patient's home, if the performance of such tests meets such conditions relating to health and safety as the Secretary may find necessary and including diagnostic mammography if conducted by a facility that has a certificate (or provisional certificate) issued under section 354 of the Public Health Service Act), diagnostic laboratory tests, and other diagnostic tests;

(4) X-ray, radium, and radioactive isotope therapy, including materials and services of technicians;

(5) surgical dressings, and splints, casts, and other devices used for reduction of fractures and dislocations;

(6) durable medical equipment;

(7) ambulance service where the use of other methods of transportation is contraindicated by the individual's condition, but, subject to section 1834(l)(14), only to the extent provided in regulations;

(8) prosthetic devices (other than dental) which replace all or part of an internal body organ (including colostomy bags and supplies directly related to colostomy care), including replacement of such devices, and including one pair of conventional eyeglasses or contact lenses furnished subsequent to each cataract surgery with insertion of an intraocular lens;

(9) leg, arm, back, and neck braces, and artificial legs, arms, and eyes, including replacements if required because of a change in the patient's physical condition;

(10) (10) (A) pneumococcal vaccine and its administration and, subject to section 4071(b) of the Omnibus Budget Reconciliation Act of 1987, influenza vaccine and its administration; and

(B) hepatitis B vaccine and its administration, furnished to an individual who is at high or intermediate risk of contracting hepatitis B (as determined by the Secretary under regulations);

(11) services of a certified registered nurse anesthetist (as defined in subsection (bb));

(12) subject to section 4072(e) of the Omnibus Budget Reconciliation Act of 1987, extra-depth shoes with inserts or custom molded shoes with inserts for an individual with diabetes, if—

(A) the physician who is managing the individual's diabetic condition (i) documents that the individual has peripheral neuropathy with evidence of callus formation, a history of pre-ulcerative calluses, a history of previous ulceration, foot deformity, or previous amputation, or poor circulation, and (ii) certifies that the individual needs such shoes under a comprehensive plan of care related to the individual's diabetic condition;

(B) the particular type of shoes are prescribed by a podiatrist or other qualified physician (as established by the Secretary); and

(C) the shoes are fitted and furnished by a podiatrist or other qualified individual (such as a pedorthist or orthotist, as established by the Secretary) who is not the physician described in subparagraph (A) (unless the Secretary finds that the physician is the only such qualified individual in the area);

(13) screening mammography (as defined in subsection (jj));

(14) screening pap smear and screening pelvic exam; and

(15) bone mass measurement (as defined in subsection (rr)). No diagnostic tests performed in any laboratory, including a laboratory that is part of a rural health clinic, or a hospital (which, for purposes of this sentence, means an institution considered a hospital for purposes of section 1814(d)) shall be included within paragraph (3) unless such laboratory—

(16) if situated in any State in which State or applicable local law provides for licensing of establishments of this nature, (A) is licensed pursuant to such law, or (B) is approved, by the agency of such State or

locality responsible for licensing establishments of this nature, as meeting the standards established for such licensing; and

(17)(A) meets the certification requirements under section 353 of the Public Health Service Act; and

(B) meets such other conditions relating to the health and safety of individuals with respect to whom such tests are performed as the Secretary may find necessary.

There shall be excluded from the diagnostic services specified in paragraph (2)(C) any item or service (except services referred to in paragraph (1)) which would not be included under subsection (b) if it were furnished to an inpatient of a hospital. None of the items and services referred to in the preceding paragraphs (other than paragraphs (1) and (2)(A)) of this subsection which are furnished to a patient of an institution which meets the definition of a hospital for purposes of section 1814(d) shall be included unless such other conditions are met as the Secretary may find necessary relating to health and safety of individuals with respect to whom such items and services are furnished.

### *Drugs and Biologicals*

(t)(1) The term "drugs" and the term "biologicals," except for purposes of subsection (m)(5) and paragraph (2), include only such drugs (including contrast agents) and biologicals, respectively, as are included (or approved for inclusion) in the United States Pharmacopoeia, the National Formulary, or the United States Homeopathic Pharmacopoeia, or in New Drugs or Accepted Dental Remedies (except for any drugs and biologicals unfavorably evaluated therein), or as are approved by the pharmacy and drug therapeutics committee (or equivalent committee) of the medical staff of the hospital furnishing such drugs and biologicals for use in such hospital.

(2)(A) For purposes of paragraph (1), the term "drugs" also includes any drugs or biologicals used in an anticancer chemotherapeutic regimen for a medically accepted indication (as described in subparagraph (B)).

(B) In subparagraph (A), the term "medically accepted indication," with respect to the use of a drug, includes any use which has been approved by the Food and Drug Administration for the drug, and includes another use of the drug if—

(i) the drug has been approved by the Food and Drug Administration; and

(ii)(I) such use is supported by one or more citations which are included (or approved for inclusion) in one or more of the following compendia: the American Hospital Formulary Service-Drug Information, the American Medical Association Drug Evaluations, the United States Pharmacopoeia-Drug Information (or its successor publications), and other authoritative compendia as identified by the Secretary, unless the Secretary has determined that the use is not medically appropriate or the use is identified as not indicated in one or more such compendia, or

(II) the carrier involved determines, based upon guidance provided by the Secretary to carriers for determining accepted uses of drugs, that such use is medically accepted based on supportive clinical evidence in peer reviewed medical literature appearing in publications which have been identified for purposes of this subclause by the Secretary.

The Secretary may revise the list of compendia in clause (ii)(I) as is appropriate for identifying medically accepted indications for drugs. On and after January 1, 2010, no compendia may be included on the list of compendia under this subparagraph unless the compendia has a publicly transparent process for evaluating therapies and for identifying potential conflicts of interests.

***Provider of Services***

(u) The term "provider of services" means a hospital, critical access hospital, skilled nursing facility, comprehensive outpatient rehabilitation facility, home health agency, hospice program, or, for purposes of section 1814(g) and section 1835(e), a fund.

***Reasonable Cost***

(v)(1)(A) The reasonable cost of any services shall be the cost actually incurred, excluding therefrom any part of incurred cost found to be unnecessary in the efficient delivery of needed health services, and shall be determined in accordance with regulations establishing the method or methods to be used, and the items to be included, in determining such costs for various types or classes of institutions, agencies, and services; except that in any case to which paragraph (2) or (3) applies, the amount of the payment determined under such paragraph with respect to the services involved shall be considered the reasonable cost of such services. In prescribing the regulations referred to in the preceding sentence, the Secretary shall consider, among other things, the principles generally applied by national organizations or established prepayment organizations (which have developed such principles) in computing the amount of payment, to be made by persons other than the recipients of services, to providers of services on account of services furnished to such recipients by such providers. Such regulations may provide for determination of the costs of services on a per diem, per unit, per capita, or other basis, may provide for using different methods in different circumstances, may provide for the use of estimates of costs of particular items or services, may provide for the establishment of limits on the direct or indirect overall incurred costs or incurred costs of specific items or services or groups of items or services to be recognized as reasonable based on estimates of the costs necessary in the efficient delivery of needed health services to individuals covered by the insurance programs established under this title, and may provide for the use of charges or a percentage of charges where this method reasonably reflects the costs. Such regulations shall (i) take into account both direct and indirect costs of providers of services (excluding therefrom any such costs, including standby costs, which are determined in accordance with regulations to be unnecessary in the efficient delivery of services covered by the insurance programs established under this title) in order that, under the methods of determining costs, the necessary costs of efficiently delivering covered services to individuals covered by the insurance programs established by this title will not be borne by individuals not so covered, and the costs with respect to individuals not so covered will not be borne by such insurance programs, and (ii) provide for the making of suitable retroactive corrective adjustments where, for a provider of services for any fiscal period, the aggregate reimbursement produced by the methods of determining costs proves to be either inadequate or excessive.

(B) In the case of extended care services, the regulations under subparagraph (A) shall not include provision for specific recognition of a return on equity capital.

(C) Where a hospital has an arrangement with a medical school under which the faculty of such school provides services at such hospital, an amount not in excess of the reasonable cost of such services to the medical school shall be included in determining the reasonable cost to the hospital of furnishing services—

(i) for which payment may be made under part A, but only if—

(I) payment for such services as furnished under such arrangement would be made under part A to the hospital had such services been furnished by the hospital, and

(II) such hospital pays to the medical school at least the reasonable cost of such services to the medical school, or

(ii) for which payment may be made under part B, but only if such hospital pays to the medical school at least the reasonable cost of such services to the medical school.

(D) Where (i) physicians furnish services which are either inpatient hospital services (including services in conjunction with the teaching programs of such hospital) by reason of paragraph (7) of subsection (b) or for which entitlement exists by reason of clause

(II) of section 1832(a)(2)(B)(i), and (ii) such hospital (or medical school under arrangement with such hospital) incurs no actual cost in the furnishing of such services, the reasonable cost of such services shall (under regulations of the Secretary) be deemed to be the cost such hospital or medical school would have incurred had it paid a salary to such physicians rendering such services approximately equivalent to the average salary paid to all physicians employed by such hospital (or if such employment does not exist, or is minimal in such hospital, by similar hospitals in a geographic area of sufficient size to assure reasonable inclusion of sufficient physicians in development of such average salary).

(E) Such regulations may, in the case of skilled nursing facilities in any State, provide for the use of rates, developed by the State in which such facilities are located, for the payment of the cost of skilled nursing facility services furnished under the State's plan approved under title XIX (and such rates may be increased by the Secretary on a class or size of institution or on a geographical basis by a percentage factor not in excess of 10 percent to take into account determinable items or services or other requirements under this title not otherwise included in the computation of such State rates), if the Secretary finds that such rates are reasonably related to (but not necessarily limited to) analyses undertaken by such State of costs of care in comparable facilities in such State. Not-withstanding the previous sentence, such regulations with respect to skilled nursing facilities shall take into account (in a manner consistent with subparagraph (A) and based on patient-days of services furnished) the costs (including the costs of services required to attain or maintain the highest practicable physical, mental, and psychosocial well-being of each resident eligible for benefits under this title) of such facilities complying with the requirements of subsections (b), (c), and (d) of section 1819 (including the costs of conducting nurse aide training and competency evaluation programs and competency evaluation programs).

(F) Such regulations shall require each provider of services (other than a fund) to make reports to the Secretary of information described in section 1121(a) in accordance with the uniform reporting system (established under such section) for that type of provider. (G)(i) In any case in which a hospital provides inpatient services to an individual that would constitute post-hospital extended care services if provided by a skilled nursing facility and a quality improvement organization (or, in the absence of such a qualified organization, the Secretary or such agent as the Secretary may designate) determines that inpatient hospital services for the individual are not medically necessary but post-hospital extended care services for the individual are medically necessary and such extended care services are not otherwise available to the individual (as determined in accordance with criteria established by the Secretary) at the time of such determination, payment for such services provided to the individual shall continue to be made under this title at the payment rate described in clause (ii) during the period in which—

(I) such post-hospital extended care services for the individual are medically necessary and not otherwise available to the individual (as so determined),

(II) inpatient hospital services for the individual are not medically necessary, and

(III) the individual is entitled to have payment made for post-hospital extended care services under this title,

except that if the Secretary determines that there is not an excess of hospital beds in such hospital and (subject to clause (iv)) there is not an excess of hospital beds in the area of such hospital, such payment shall be made (during such period) on the basis of the amount otherwise payable under part A with respect to inpatient hospital services.

(ii)(I) Except as provided in subclause (II), the payment rate referred to in clause (i) is a rate equal to the estimated adjusted State-wide average rate per patient-day paid for services provided in skilled nursing facilities under the State plan approved under title XIX for the State in which such hospital is located, or, if the State in which the hospital is located does not have a State plan approved under title XIX, the estimated adjusted State-wide average allowable costs per patient-day for extended care services under this title in that State.

(II) If a hospital has a unit which is a skilled nursing facility, the payment rate referred to in clause (i) for the hospital is a rate equal to the lesser of the rate described in subclause (I) or the allowable costs in effect under this title for extended care services provided to patients of such unit.

(iii) Any day on which an individual receives inpatient services for which payment is made under this subparagraph shall, for purposes of this Act (other than this subparagraph), be deemed to be a day on which the individual received inpatient hospital services.

(iv) In determining under clause (i), in the case of a public hospital, whether or not there is an excess of hospital beds in the area of such hospital, such determination shall be made on the basis of only the public hospitals (including the hospital) which are in the area of the hospital and which are under common ownership with that hospital.

(H) In determining such reasonable cost with respect to home health agencies, the Secretary may not include—

(i) any costs incurred in connection with bonding or establishing an escrow account by any such agency as a result of the surety bond requirement described in subsection (o)(7) and the financial security requirement described in subsection (o)(8);

(ii) in the case of home health agencies to which the surety bond requirement described in subsection (o)(7) and the financial security requirement described in subsection (o)(8) apply, any costs attributed to interest charged such an agency in connection with amounts borrowed by the agency to repay over-payments made under this title to the agency, except that such costs may be included in reasonable cost if the Secretary determines that the agency was acting in good faith in borrowing the amounts;

(iii) in the case of contracts entered into by a home health agency after the date of the enactment of this subparagraph for the purpose of having services furnished for or on behalf of such agency, any cost incurred by such agency pursuant to any such contract which is entered into for a period exceeding five years; and

(iv) in the case of contracts entered into by a home health agency before the date of the enactment of this subparagraph for the purpose of having services furnished for or on behalf of such agency, any cost incurred by such agency pursuant to any such contract, which determines the amount payable by the home health agency on the basis of a percentage of the agency's reimbursement or claim for reimbursement for services furnished by the agency, to the extent that such cost exceeds the reasonable value of the services furnished on behalf of such agency.

(I) In determining such reasonable cost, the Secretary may not include any costs incurred by a provider with respect to any services furnished in connection with matters for which payment may be made under this title and furnished pursuant to a contract between the provider and any of its subcontractors which is entered into after the date of the enactment of this subparagraph and the value or cost of which is $10,000 or more over a twelve-month period unless the contract contains a clause to the effect that—

(i) until the expiration of four years after the furnishing of such services pursuant to such contract, the subcontractor shall make available, upon written request by the Secretary, or upon request by the Comptroller General, or any of their duly authorized representatives, the contract, and books, documents and records of such subcontractor that are necessary to certify the nature and extent of such costs, and

(ii) if the subcontractor carries out any of the duties of the contract through a subcontract, with a value or cost of $10,000 or more over a twelve-month period, with a related organization, such subcontract shall contain a clause to the effect that until the expiration of four years after the furnishing of such services pursuant to such subcontract, the related organization shall make available, upon written request by the Secretary, or upon request by the Comptroller General, or any of their duly authorized representatives, the subcontract, and books, documents and records of such organization that are necessary to verify the nature and extent of such costs.

The Secretary shall prescribe in regulation criteria and procedures which the Secretary shall use in obtaining access to books, documents, and records under clauses required in contracts and subcontracts under this subparagraph.

(J) Such regulations may not provide for any inpatient routine salary cost differential as a reimbursable cost for hospitals and skilled nursing facilities.

(K)(i) The Secretary shall issue regulations that provide, to the extent feasible, for the establishment of limitations on the amount of any costs or charges that shall be considered reasonable with respect to services provided on an outpatient basis by hospitals (other than bona fide emergency services as defined in clause (ii)) or clinics (other than rural health clinics), which are reimbursed on a cost basis or on the basis of cost related charges, and by physicians utilizing such outpatient facilities. Such limitations shall be reasonably related to the charges in the same area for similar services provided in physicians' offices. Such regulations shall provide for exceptions to such limitations in cases where similar services are not generally available in physicians' offices in the area to individuals entitled to benefits under this title.

(ii) For purposes of clause (i), the term "bona fide emergency services" means services provided in a hospital emergency room after the sudden onset of a medical condition manifesting itself by acute symptoms of sufficient severity (including severe pain) such that the absence of immediate medical attention could reasonably be expected to result in—

(I) placing the patient's health in serious jeopardy;

(II) serious impairment to bodily functions; or

(III) serious dysfunction of any bodily organ or part.

(L)(i) The Secretary, in determining the amount of the payments that may be made under this title with respect to services furnished by home health agencies, may not recognize as reasonable (in the efficient delivery of such services) costs for the provision of such services by an agency to the extent these costs exceed (on the aggregate for the agency) for cost reporting periods beginning on or after—

(I) July 1, 1985, and before July 1, 1986, 120 percent of the mean of the labor-related and nonlabor per visit costs for free-standing home health agencies,

(II) July 1, 1986, and before July 1, 1987, 115 percent of such mean,

(III) July 1, 1987, and before October 1, 1997, 112 percent of such mean,

(IV) October 1, 1997, and before October 1, 1998, 105 percent of the median of the labor-related and nonlabor per visit costs for freestanding home health agencies, or

(V) October 1, 1998, 106 percent of such median.

(ii) Effective for cost reporting periods beginning on or after July 1, 1986, such limitations shall be applied on an aggregate basis for the agency, rather than on a discipline specific basis. The Secretary may provide for such exemptions and exceptions to such limitation as he deems appropriate.

(iii) Not later than July 1, 1991, and annually thereafter (but not for cost reporting periods beginning on or after July 1, 1994, and before July 1, 1996, or on or after July 1, 1997, and before October 1, 1997), the Secretary shall establish limits under this subparagraph for cost reporting periods beginning on or after such date by utilizing the area wage index applicable under section 1886(d)(3)(E) and determined using the survey of the most recent available wages and wage-related costs of hospitals located in the geographic area in which the home health service is furnished (determined without regard to whether such hospitals have been reclassified to a new geographic area pursuant to section 1886(d)(8)(B), a decision of the Medicare Geographic Classification Review Board under section 1886(d)(10), or a decision of the Secretary).

(iv) In establishing limits under this subparagraph for cost reporting periods beginning after September 30, 1997, the Secretary shall not take into account any changes in the home health market basket, as determined by the Secretary, with respect to cost reporting periods which began on or after July 1, 1994, and before July 1, 1996.

(v) For services furnished by home health agencies for cost reporting periods beginning on or after October 1, 1997, subject to clause (viii)(I), the Secretary shall provide for an interim system of limits. Payment shall not exceed the costs determined under the preceding provisions of this subparagraph or, if lower, the product of—

(I) an agency-specific per beneficiary annual limitation calculated based 75 percent on 98 percent of the reasonable costs (including nonroutine medical supplies) for the agency's 12-month cost reporting period ending during fiscal year 1994, and based 25 percent on 98 percent of the standardized regional average of such costs for the agency's census division, as applied to such agency, for cost reporting periods ending during fiscal year 1994, such costs updated by the home health market basket index; and

(II) the agency's unduplicated census count of patients (entitled to benefits under this title) for the cost reporting period subject to the limitation.

(vi) For services furnished by home health agencies for cost reporting periods beginning on or after October 1, 1997, the following rules apply:

(I) For new providers and those providers without a 12-month cost reporting period ending in fiscal year 1994 subject to clauses (viii)(II) and (viii)(III), the per beneficiary limitation shall be equal to the median of these limits (or the Secretary's best estimates thereof) applied to other home health agencies as determined by the Secretary. A home health agency that has altered its corporate structure or name shall not be considered a new provider for this purpose.

(II) For beneficiaries who use services furnished by more than one home health agency, the per beneficiary limitations shall be prorated among the agencies.

(vii)(I) Not later than January 1, 1998, the Secretary shall establish per visit limits applicable for fiscal year 1998, and not later than April 1, 1998, the Secretary shall establish per beneficiary limits under clause (v)(I) for fiscal year 1998.

(II) Not later than August 1 of each year (beginning in 1998) the Secretary shall establish the limits applicable under this subparagraph for services furnished during the fiscal year beginning October 1 of the year.

(viii)(I) In the case of a provider with a 12-month cost reporting period ending in fiscal year 1994, if the limit imposed under clause

(v) (determined without regard to this subclause) for a cost reporting period beginning during or after fiscal year 1999 is less than the median described in clause (vi)(I) (but determined as if any reference in clause (v) to "98 percent" were a reference to "100 percent"), the limit otherwise imposed under clause (v) for such provider and period shall be increased by ⅓ of such difference.

(II) Subject to subclause (IV), for new providers and those providers without a 12-month cost reporting period ending in fiscal year 1994, but for which the first cost reporting period begins before fiscal year 1999, for cost reporting periods beginning during or after fiscal year 1999, the per beneficiary limitation described in clause (vi)(I) shall be equal to the median described in such clause (determined as if any reference in clause (v) to "98 percent" were a reference to "100 percent").

(III) Subject to subclause (IV), in the case of a new provider for which the first cost reporting period begins during or after fiscal year 1999, the limitation applied under clause (vi)(I) (but only with respect to such provider) shall be equal to 75 percent of the median described in clause (vi)(I).

(IV) In the case of a new provider or a provider without a 12-month cost reporting period ending in fiscal year 1994, subclause

(II) shall apply, instead of subclause (III), to a home health agency which filed an application for home health agency provider status under this title before September 15, 1998, or which was approved as a branch of its parent agency before such date and becomes a subunit of the parent agency or a separate agency on or after such date.

(V) Each of the amounts specified in subclauses (I) through (III) are such amounts as adjusted under clause (iii) to reflect variations in wages among different areas.

(ix) Notwithstanding the per beneficiary limit under clause (viii), if the limit imposed under clause (v) (determined without regard to this clause) for a cost reporting period beginning during or after fiscal year 2000 is less than the median described in clause (vi)(I) (but determined as if any reference in clause (v) to "98 percent" were a reference to "100 percent"), the limit otherwise imposed under clause (v) for such provider and period shall be increased by 2 percent.

(x) Notwithstanding any other provision of this subparagraph, in updating any limit under this subparagraph by a home health market basket index for cost reporting periods beginning during each of fiscal years 2000, 2002, and 2003, the update otherwise provided shall be reduced by 1.1 percentage points. With respect to cost reporting periods beginning during fiscal year 2001, the update to any limit under this subparagraph shall be the home health market basket index.

(M) Such regulations shall provide that costs respecting care provided by a provider of services, pursuant to an assurance under title VI or XVI of the Public Health Service Act that the provider will make available a reasonable volume of services to persons unable to pay therefor, shall not be allowable as reasonable costs.

(N) In determining such reasonable costs, costs incurred for activities directly related to influencing employees respecting unionization may not be included.

(O)(i) In establishing an appropriate allowance for depreciation and for interest on capital indebtedness with respect to an asset of a provider of services which has undergone a change of ownership, such regulations shall provide, except as provided in clause (iii), that the valuation of the asset after such change of ownership shall be the historical cost of the asset, as recognized under this title, less depreciation allowed, to the owner of record as of the date of enactment of the Balanced Budget Act of 1997 (or, in the case of an asset not in existence as of that date, the first owner of record of the asset after that date).

(ii) Such regulations shall not recognize, as reasonable in the provision of health care services, costs (including legal fees, accounting and administrative costs, travel costs, and the costs of feasibility studies) attributable to the negotiation or settlement of the sale or purchase of any capital asset (by acquisition or merger) for which any payment has previously been made under this title.

(iii)In the case of the transfer of a hospital from ownership by a State to ownership by a nonprofit corporation without monetary consideration, the basis for capital allowances to the new owner shall be the book value of the hospital to the State at the time of the transfer.

(P) If such regulations provide for the payment for a return on equity capital (other than with respect to costs of inpatient hospital services), the rate of return to be recognized, for determining the reasonable cost of services furnished in a cost reporting period, shall be equal to the average of the rates of interest, for each of the months any part of which is included in the period, on obligations issued for purchase by the Federal Hospital Insurance Trust Fund.

(Q) Except as otherwise explicitly authorized, the Secretary is not authorized to limit the rate of increase on allowable costs of approved medical educational activities.

(R) In determining such reasonable cost, costs incurred by a provider of services representing a beneficiary in an unsuccessful appeal of a determination described in section 1869(b) shall not be allowable as reasonable costs.

(S)(i) Such regulations shall not include provision for specific recognition of any return on equity capital with respect to hospital outpatient departments.

(ii)(I) Such regulations shall provide that, in determining the amount of the payments that may be made under this title with respect to all the capital-related costs of outpatient hospital services, the Secretary shall reduce the amounts of such payments otherwise established under this title by 15 percent for payments attributable to portions of cost reporting periods occurring during fiscal year 1990, by 15 percent for payments attributable to portions of cost reporting periods occurring during fiscal year 1991, and by 10 percent for payments attributable to portions of cost reporting periods occurring during fiscal years 1992 through 1999 and until the first date that the prospective payment system under section 1833(t) is implemented.

(II) The Secretary shall reduce the reasonable cost of outpatient hospital services (other than the capital-related costs of such services) otherwise determined pursuant to section 1833(a)(2)(B)(i)(I) by 5.8 percent for payments attributable to portions of cost reporting periods occurring during fiscal years 1991 through 1999 and until the first date that the prospective payment system under section 1833(t) is implemented.

(III) Subclauses (I) and (II) shall not apply to payments with respect to the costs of hospital outpatient services provided by any hospital that is a sole community hospital (as defined in section 1886(d)(5)(D)(iii)) or a critical access hospital (as defined in section 1861(mm)(1)).

(IV) In applying subclauses (I) and (II) to services for which payment is made on the basis of a blend amount under section 1833(i)(3)(A)(ii) or 1833(n)(1)(A)(ii), the costs reflected in the amounts described in sections 1833(i)(3)(B)(i)(I) and 1833(n)(1)(B)(i)(I), respectively, shall be reduced in accordance with such subclause.

(T) In determining such reasonable costs for hospitals, no reduction in copayments under section 1833(t)(8)(B) shall be treated as a bad debt and the amount of bad debts otherwise treated as allowable costs which are attributable to the deductibles and coinsurance amounts under this title shall be reduced—

(i) for cost reporting periods beginning during fiscal year 1998, by 25 percent of such amount otherwise allowable,

(ii) for cost reporting periods beginning during fiscal year 1999, by 40 percent of such amount otherwise allowable,

(iii) for cost reporting periods beginning during fiscal year 2000, by 45 percent of such amount otherwise allowable,

(iv) for cost reporting periods beginning during fiscal years 2001 through 2012, by 30 percent of such amount otherwise allowable, and

(v) for cost reporting periods beginning during fiscal year 2013 or a subsequent fiscal year, by 35 percent of such amount otherwise allowable.

(U) In determining the reasonable cost of ambulance services (as described in subsection (s)(7)) provided during fiscal year 1998, during fiscal year 1999, and during so much of fiscal year 2000 as precedes January 1, 2000, the Secretary shall not recognize the costs per trip in excess of costs recognized as reasonable for ambulance services provided on a per trip basis during the previous fiscal year (after application of this subparagraph), increased by the percentage increase in the consumer price index for all urban consumers (U.S. city average) as estimated by the Secretary for the 12-month period ending with the midpoint of the fiscal year involved reduced by 1.0 percentage point. For ambulance services provided after June 30, 1998, the Secretary may provide that claims for such services must include a code (or codes) under a uniform coding system specified by the Secretary that identifies the services furnished.

(V) In determining such reasonable costs for skilled nursing facilities and (beginning with respect to cost reporting periods beginning during fiscal year 2013) for covered skilled nursing services described in section 1888(e)(2)(A) furnished by hospital providers of extended care services (as described in section 1883), the amount of bad debts otherwise treated as allowed costs which are attributable to the coinsurance amounts under this title for individuals who are entitled to benefits under part A and—

(i) are not described in section 1935(c)(6)(A)(ii) shall be reduced by—

(I) for cost reporting periods beginning on or after October 1, 2005, but before fiscal year 2013, 30 percent of such amount otherwise allowable; and

(II) for cost reporting periods beginning during fiscal year 2013 or a subsequent fiscal year, by 35 percent of such amount otherwise allowable.

(ii) are described in such section—

(I) for cost reporting periods beginning on or after October 1, 2005, but before fiscal year 2013, shall not be reduced;

(II) for cost reporting periods beginning during fiscal year 2013, shall be reduced by 12 percent of such amount otherwise allowable;

(III) for cost reporting periods beginning during fiscal year 2014, shall be reduced by 24 percent of such amount otherwise allowable; and

(IV) for cost reporting periods beginning during a subsequent fiscal year, shall be reduced by 35 percent of such amount otherwise allowable.

(W)(i) In determining such reasonable costs for providers described in clause (ii), the amount of bad debts otherwise treated as allowable costs which are attributable to deductibles and coinsurance amounts under this title shall be reduced—

(I) for cost reporting periods beginning during fiscal year 2013, by 12 percent of such amount otherwise allowable;

(II) for cost reporting periods beginning during fiscal year 2014, by 24 percent of such amount otherwise allowable; and

(III) for cost reporting periods beginning during a subsequent fiscal year, by 35 percent of such amount otherwise allowable.

(ii) A provider described in this clause is a provider of services not described in subparagraph (T) or (V), a supplier, or any other type of entity that receives payment for bad debts under the authority under subparagraph (A).

(2)(A) If the bed and board furnished as part of inpatient hospital services (including inpatient tuberculosis hospital services and in-patient psychiatric hospital services) or post-hospital extended care services is in accommodations more expensive than semi-private accommodations, the amount taken into account for purposes of payment under this title with respect to such services may not exceed the amount that would be taken into account with respect to such services if furnished in such semi-private accommodations un- less the more expensive accommodations were required for medical reasons.

(B) Where a provider of services which has an agreement in effect under this title furnishes to an individual items or services which are in excess of or more expensive than the items or services with respect to which payment may be made under part A or part B, as the case may be, the Secretary shall take into account for purposes of payment to such provider of services only the items or services with respect to which such payment may be made.

(3) If the bed and board furnished as part of inpatient hospital services (including inpatient tuberculosis hospital services and inpatient psychiatric hospital services) or post-hospital extended care services is in accommodations other than, but not more expensive than, semi-private accommodations and the use of such other accommodations rather than semi-private accommodations was neither at the request of the patient nor for a reason which the Secretary determines is consistent with the purposes of this title, the amount of the payment with respect to such bed and board under part A shall be the amount otherwise payable under this title for such bed and board furnished in semi-private accommodations minus the difference between the charge customarily made by the hospital or skilled nursing facility for bed and board in semi-private accommodations and the charge customarily made by it for bed and board in the accommodations furnished.

(4) If a provider of services furnishes items or services to an individual which are in excess of or more expensive than the items or services determined to be necessary in the efficient delivery of needed health services and charges are imposed for such more expensive items or services under the authority granted in section 1866(a)(2)(B)(ii), the amount of payment with respect to such items or services otherwise due such provider in any fiscal period shall be reduced to the extent that such payment plus such charges exceed the cost actually incurred for such items or services in the fiscal period in which such charges are imposed.

(5)(A) Where physical therapy services, occupational therapy services, speech therapy services, or other therapy services or services of other health-related personnel (other than physicians) are furnished under an arrangement with a provider of services or other organization, specified in the first sentence of subsection (p) (including through the operation of subsection (g)) the amount included in any payment to such provider or other organization under this title as the reasonable cost of such services (as furnished under such arrangements) shall not exceed an amount equal to the salary which would reasonably have been paid for such services (together with any additional costs that would have been incurred by the provider or other organization) to the person performing them if they had been performed in an employment relationship with such provider or other organization (rather than under such arrangement) plus the cost of such other expenses (including a reasonable allowance for traveltime and other reasonable types of expense related to any differences in acceptable methods of organization for the provision of such therapy) incurred by such person, as the Secretary may in regulations determine to be appropriate.

(B) Notwithstanding the provisions of subparagraph (A), if a provider of services or other organization specified in the first sentence of section 1861(p) requires the services of a therapist on a limited part-time basis, or only to perform intermittent services, the Secretary may make payment on the basis of a reasonable rate per unit of service, even though such rate is greater per unit of time than salary related amounts, where he finds that such greater payment is, in the aggregate, less than the amount that would have been paid if such organization had employed a therapist on a full- or part-time salary basis.

(6) For purposes of this subsection, the term "semi-private accommodations" means two-bed, three-bed, or four-bed accommodations.

(7)(A) For limitation on Federal participation for capital expenditures which are out of conformity with a comprehensive plan of a State or areawide planning agency, see section 1122.

(B) For further limitations on reasonable cost and determination of payment amounts for operating costs of inpatient hospital services and waivers for certain States, see section 1886.

(C) For provisions restricting payment for provider-based physicians' services and for payments under certain percentage arrangements, see section 1887.

(D) For further limitations on reasonable cost and determination of payment amounts for routine service costs of skilled nursing facilities, see subsections (a) through (c) of section 1888.

(8) ITEMS UNRELATED TO PATIENT CARE.—Reasonable costs do not include costs for the following—

(i) entertainment, including tickets to sporting and other entertainment events;

(ii) gifts or donations;

(iii) personal use of motor vehicles;

(iv) costs for fines and penalties resulting from violations of Federal, State, or local laws; and

(v) education expenses for spouses or other dependents of providers of services, their employees or contractors.

### *Arrangements for Certain Services*

(w)(1) The term "arrangements" is limited to arrangements under which receipt of payment by the hospital, critical access hospital, skilled nursing facility, home health agency, or hospice program (whether in its own right or as agent), with respect to services for which an individual is entitled to have payment made under this title, discharges the liability of such individual or any other person to pay for the services.

(2) Utilization review activities conducted, in accordance with the requirements of the program established under part B of title XI of the Social Security Act with respect to services furnished by a hospital or critical access hospital to patients insured under part A of this title or entitled to have payment made for such services under part B of this title or under a State plan approved under title XIX, by a quality improvement organization designated for the area in which such hospital or critical

access hospital is located shall be deemed to have been conducted pursuant to arrangements between such hospital or critical access hospital and such organization under which such hospital or critical access hospital is obligated to pay to such organization, as a condition of receiving payment for hospital or critical access hospital services so furnished under this part or under such a State plan, such amount as is reasonably incurred and requested (as determined under regulations of the Secretary) by such organization in conducting such review activities with respect to services furnished by such hospital or critical access hospital to such patients.

***State and United States***

(x) The terms "State" and "United States" have the meaning given to them by subsections (h) and (i), respectively, of section 210.

***Extended Care in Religious Nonmedical Health Care Institutions***

(y)(1) The term "skilled nursing facility" also includes a religious nonmedical health care institution (as defined in subsection (ss)(1)), but only (except for purposes of subsection (a)(2)) with respect to items and services ordinarily furnished by such an institution to inpatients, and payment may be made with respect to services provided by or in such an institution only to such extent and under such conditions, limitations, and requirements (in addition to or in lieu of the conditions, limitations, and requirements otherwise applicable) as may be provided in regulations consistent with section 1821.

(2) Notwithstanding any other provision of this title, payment under part A may not be made for services furnished an individual in a skilled nursing facility to which paragraph (1) applies unless such individual elects, in accordance with regulations, for a spell of illness to have such services treated as post-hospital extended care services for purposes of such part; and payment under part A may not be made for post-hospital extended care services—

(A) furnished an individual during such spell of illness in a skilled nursing facility to which paragraph (1) applies after—

(i) such services have been furnished to him in such a facility for 30 days during such spell, or

(ii) such services have been furnished to him during such spell in a skilled nursing facility to which such paragraph does not apply; or

(B) furnished an individual during such spell of illness in a skilled nursing facility to which paragraph (1) does not apply after such services have been furnished to him during such spell in a skilled nursing facility to which such paragraph applies.

(3) The amount payable under part A for post-hospital extended care services furnished an individual during any spell of illness in a skilled nursing facility to which paragraph (1) applies shall be reduced by a coinsurance amount equal to one-eighth of the inpatient hospital deductible for each day before the 31st day on which he is furnished such services in such a facility during such spell (and the reduction under this paragraph shall be in lieu of any reduction under section 1813(a)(3)).

(4) For purposes of subsection (i), the determination of whether services furnished by or in an institution described in paragraph

(1) constitute post-hospital extended care services shall be made in accordance with and subject to such conditions, limitations, and requirements as may be provided in regulations.

### *Institutional Planning*

(z) An overall plan and budget of a hospital, skilled nursing facility, comprehensive outpatient rehabilitation facility, or home health agency shall be considered sufficient if it—

(1) provides for an annual operating budget which includes all anticipated income and expenses related to items which would, under generally accepted accounting principles, be considered income and expense items (except that nothing in this paragraph shall require that there be prepared, in connection with any budget, an item-by-item identification of the components of each type of anticipated expenditure or income);

(2)(A) provides for a capital expenditures plan for at least a 3-year period (including the year to which the operating budget described in paragraph (1) is applicable) which includes and identifies in detail the anticipated sources of financing for, and the objectives of, each anticipated expenditure in excess of $600,000 (or such lesser amount as may be established by the State under section 1122(g)(1) in which the hospital is located) related to the acquisition of land, the improvement of land, buildings, and equipment, and the replacement, modernization, and expansion of the buildings and equipment which would, under generally accepted accounting principles, be considered capital items;

(B) provides that such plan is submitted to the agency designated under section 1122(b), or if no such agency is designated, to the appropriate health planning agency in the State (but this subparagraph shall not apply in the case of a facility exempt from review under section 1122 by reason of section 1122(j));

(3) provides for review and updating at least annually; and

(4) is prepared, under the direction of the governing body of the institution or agency, by a committee consisting of representatives of the governing body, the administrative staff, and the medical staff (if any) of the institution or agency.

### *Rural Health Clinic Services and Federally Qualified Health Center Services*

(aa)(1) The term “rural health clinic services” means —

(A) physicians’ services and such services and supplies as are covered under section 1861(s)(2)(A) if furnished as an incident to a physician’s professional service and items and services described in section 1861(s)(10),

(B) such services furnished by a physician assistant or a nurse practitioner (as defined in paragraph (5)), by a clinical psychologist (as defined by the Secretary) or by a clinical social worker (as defined in subsection (hh)(1)), and such services and supplies furnished as an incident to his service as would otherwise be covered if furnished by a physician or as an incident to a physician’s service, and

(C) in the case of a rural health clinic located in an area in which there exists a shortage of home health agencies, part-time or intermittent nursing care and related medical supplies (other than drugs and biologicals)

furnished by a registered professional nurse or licensed practical nurse to a homebound individual under a written plan of treatment (i) established and periodically reviewed by a physician described in paragraph (2)(B), or (ii) established by a nurse practitioner or physician assistant and periodically reviewed and approved by a physician described in paragraph (2)(B), when furnished to an individual as an outpatient of a rural health clinic.

(2) The term "rural health clinic" means a facility which —

(A) is primarily engaged in furnishing to outpatients services described in subparagraphs (A) and (B) of paragraph (1);

(B) in the case of a facility which is not a physician-directed clinic, has an arrangement (consistent with the provisions of State and local law relative to the practice, performance, and delivery of health services) with one or more physicians (as defined in subsection (r)(1)) under which provision is made for the periodic review by such physicians of covered services furnished by physician assistants and nurse practitioners, the supervision and guidance by such physicians of physician assistants and nurse practitioners, the preparation by such physicians of such medical orders for care and treatment of clinic patients as may be necessary, and the availability of such physicians for such referral of and consultation for patients as is necessary and for advice and assistance in the management of medical emergencies; and, in the case of a physician-directed clinic, has one or more of its staff physicians perform the activities accomplished through such an arrangement;

(C) maintains clinical records on all patients;

(D) has arrangements with one or more hospitals, having agreements in effect under section 1866, for the referral and admission of patients requiring inpatient services or such diagnostic or other specialized services as are not available at the clinic;

(E) has written policies, which are developed with the advice of (and with provision for review of such policies from time to time by) a group of professional personnel, including one or more physicians and one or more physician assistants or nurse practitioners, to govern those services described in paragraph

(1) which it furnishes;

(F) has a physician, physician assistant, or nurse practitioner responsible for the execution of policies described in sub-paragraph (E) and relating to the provision of the clinic's services;

(G) directly provides routine diagnostic services, including clinical laboratory services, as prescribed in regulations by the Secretary, and has prompt access to additional diagnostic services from facilities meeting requirements under this title;

(H) in compliance with State and Federal law, has available for administering to patients of the clinic at least such drugs and biologicals as are determined by the Secretary to be necessary for the treatment of emergency cases (as defined in regulations) and has appropriate procedures or arrangements for storing, administering, and dispensing any drugs and biologicals;

(I) has a quality assessment and performance improvement program, and appropriate procedures for review of utilization of clinic services, as the Secretary may specify;

() has a nurse practitioner, a physician assistant, or a certified nurse-midwife (as defined in subsection (gg)) available to furnish patient care services not less than 50 percent of the time the clinic operates; and

(K) meets such other requirements as the Secretary may find necessary in the interest of the health and safety of the individuals who are furnished services by the clinic.

For the purposes of this title, such term includes only a facility which (i) is located in an area that is not an urbanized area (as defined by the Bureau of the Census) and in which there are insufficient numbers of needed health care practitioners (as determined by the Secretary), and that, within the previous 4-year period, has been designated by the chief executive officer of the State and certified by the Secretary as an area with a shortage of personal health services or designated by the Secretary either (I) as an area with a shortage of personal health services under section 330(b)(3) or 1302(7) of the Public Health Service Act, (II) as a health professional shortage area described in section 332(a)(1)(A) of that Act because of its shortage of primary medical care manpower, (III) as a high impact area described in section 329(a)(5) of that Act, of (IV) as an area which includes a population group which the Secretary determines has a health manpower shortage under section 332(a)(1)(B) of that Act, (ii) has filed an agreement with the Secretary by which it agrees not to charge any individual or other person for items or services for which such individual is entitled to have payment made under this title, except for the amount of any deductible or coinsurance amount imposed with respect to such items or services (not in excess of the amount customarily charged for such items and services by such clinic), pursuant to subsections

(a) and (b) of section 1833, (iii) employs a physician assistant or nurse practitioner, and (iv) is not a rehabilitation agency or a facility which is primarily for the care and treatment of mental diseases. A facility that is in operation and qualifies as a rural health clinic under this title or title XIX and that subsequently fails to satisfy the requirement of clause (i) shall be considered, for purposes of this title and title XIX, as still satisfying the requirement of such clause if it is determined, in accordance with criteria established by the Secretary in regulations, to be essential to the delivery of primary care services that would otherwise be unavailable in the geographic area served by the clinic. If a State agency has determined under section 1864(a) that a facility is a rural health clinic and the facility has applied to the Secretary for approval as such a clinic, the Secretary shall notify the facility of the Secretary's approval or disapproval not later than 60 days after the date of the State agency determination or the application (whichever is later).

(3) The term "Federally qualified health center services" means—

(A) services of the type described in subparagraphs (A) through (C) of paragraph (1) and preventive services (as defined in section 1861(ddd)(3)); and

(B) preventive primary health services that a center is required to provide under section 330 of the Public Health Service Act, when furnished to an individual as an outpatient of a Federally qualified health center by the center or by a health care professional under contract with the center and, for this purpose, any reference to a rural health clinic or a physician described in paragraph (2)(B) is deemed a reference to a Federally qualified health center or a physician at the center, respectively.

(4) The term "Federally qualified health center" means an entity which—

(A)(i) is receiving a grant under section 330 of the Public Health Service Act, or

(ii)(I) is receiving funding from such a grant under a contract with the recipient of such a grant, and (II) meets the requirements to receive a grant under section 330 of such Act;

(B) based on the recommendation of the Health Resources and Services Administration within the Public Health Service, is determined by the Secretary to meet the requirements for receiving such a grant;

(C) was treated by the Secretary, for purposes of part B, as a comprehensive Federally funded health center as of January 1, 1990; or

(D) is an outpatient health program or facility operated by a tribe or tribal organization under the Indian Self-Determination Act or by an urban Indian organization receiving funds under title V of the Indian Health Care Improvement Act.

(5)(A) The term "physician assistant" and the term "nurse practitioner" mean, for purposes of this title, a physician assistant or nurse practitioner who performs such services as such individual is legally authorized to perform (in the State in which the individual performs such services) in accordance with State law (or the State regulatory mechanism provided by State law), and who meets such training, education, and experience requirements (or any combination thereof) as the Secretary may prescribe in regulations.

(B) The term "clinical nurse specialist" means, for purposes of this title, an individual who—

(i) is a registered nurse and is licensed to practice nursing in the State in which the clinical nurse specialist services are performed; and

(ii) holds a master's degree in a defined clinical area of nursing from an accredited educational institution.

(6) The term "collaboration" means a process in which a nurse practitioner works with a physician to deliver health care services within the scope of the practitioner's professional expertise, with medical direction and appropriate supervision as provided for in jointly developed

guidelines or other mechanisms as defined by the law of the State in which the services are performed.

(7)(A) The Secretary shall waive for a 1-year period the requirements of paragraph (2) that a rural health clinic employ a physician assistant, nurse practitioner or certified nurse midwife or that such clinic require such providers to furnish services at least 50 percent of the time that the clinic operates for any facility that requests such waiver if the facility demonstrates that the facility has been unable, despite reasonable efforts, to hire a physician assistant, nurse practitioner, or certified nurse-midwife in the previous 90-day period.

(B) The Secretary may not grant such a waiver under subparagraph (A) to a facility if the request for the waiver is made less than 6 months after the date of the expiration of any previous such waiver for the facility, or if the facility has not yet been determined to meet the requirements (including subparagraph (J) of the first sentence of paragraph (2)) of a rural health clinic.

(C) A waiver which is requested under this paragraph shall be deemed granted unless such request is denied by the Secretary within 60 days after the date such request is received.

### *Services of a Certified Registered Nurse Anesthetist*

(bb)(1) The term "services of a certified registered nurse anesthetist" means anesthesia services and related care furnished by a certified registered nurse anesthetist (as defined in paragraph (2)) which the nurse anesthetist is legally authorized to perform as such by the State in which the services are furnished.

(2) The term "certified registered nurse anesthetist" means a certified registered nurse anesthetist licensed by the State who meets such education, training, and other requirements relating to anesthesia services and related care as the Secretary may prescribe. In prescribing such requirements the Secretary may use the same requirements as those established by a national organization for the certification of nurse anesthetists. Such term also includes, as prescribed by the Secretary, an anesthesiologist assistant.

***Comprehensive Outpatient Rehabilitation Facility Services***

(cc)(1) The term "comprehensive outpatient rehabilitation facility services" means the following items and services furnished by a physician or other qualified professional personnel (as defined in regulations by the Secretary) to an individual who is an outpatient of a comprehensive outpatient rehabilitation facility under a plan (for furnishing such items and services to such individual) established and periodically reviewed by a physician—

(A) physicians' services;

(B) physical therapy, occupational therapy, speech-language pathology services, and respiratory therapy;

(C) prosthetic and orthotic devices, including testing, fitting, or training in the use of prosthetic and orthotic devices;

(D) social and psychological services;

(E) nursing care provided by or under the supervision of a registered professional nurse;

(F) drugs and biologicals which cannot, as determined in accordance with regulations, be self-administered;

(G) supplies and durable medical equipment; and

(H) such other items and services as are medically necessary for the rehabilitation of the patient and are ordinarily furnished by comprehensive outpatient rehabilitation facilities, excluding, however, any item or service if it would not be included under subsection (b) if furnished to an inpatient of a hospital. In the case of physical therapy, occupational therapy, and speech pathology services, there shall be no requirement that the item or service be furnished at any single fixed location if the item or service is furnished pursuant to such plan and payments are not otherwise made for the item or service under this title.

(2) The term "comprehensive outpatient rehabilitation facility" means a facility which—

(A) is primarily engaged in providing (by or under the supervision of physicians) diagnostic, therapeutic, and restorative services to outpatients for the rehabilitation of injured, disabled, or sick persons;

(B) provides at least the following comprehensive outpatient rehabilitation services: (i) physicians' services (rendered by physicians, as defined in section 1861(r)(1), who are available at the facility on a full- or part-time basis); (ii) physical therapy; and (iii) social or psychological services;

(C) maintains clinical records on all patients;

(D) has policies established by a group of professional personnel (associated with the facility), including one or more physicians defined in subsection (r)(1) to govern the comprehensive outpatient rehabilitation services it furnishes, and provides for the carrying out of such policies by a full- or part-time physician referred to in subparagraph (B)(i);

(E) has a requirement that every patient must be under the care of a physician;

(F) in the case of a facility in any State in which State or applicable local law provides for the licensing of facilities of this nature (i) is licensed pursuant to such law, or (ii) is approved by the agency of such State or locality, responsible for licensing facilities of this nature, as meeting the standards established for such licensing;

(G) has in effect a utilization review plan in accordance with regulations prescribed by the Secretary;

(H) has in effect an overall plan and budget that meets the requirements of subsection (z);

(I) provides the Secretary on a continuing basis with a surety bond in a form specified by the Secretary and in an amount that is not less than $50,000; and

(J) meets such other conditions of participation as the Secretary may find necessary in the interest of the health and safety of individuals who are furnished services by such facility, including conditions concerning qualifications of personnel in these facilities.

The Secretary may waive the requirement of a surety bond under subparagraph (I) in the case of a facility that provides a comparable surety bond under State law.

***Hospice Care; Hospice Program***

(dd)(1) The term "hospice care" means the following items and services provided to a terminally ill individual by, or by others under arrangements made by, a hospice program under a written plan (for providing such care to such individual) established and periodically reviewed by the individual's attending physician and by the medical director (and by the interdisciplinary group described in paragraph (2)(B)) of the program—

(A) nursing care provided by or under the supervision of a registered professional nurse,

(B) physical or occupational therapy, or speech-language pathology services,

(C) medical social services under the direction of a physician,

(D)(i) services of a home health aide who has successfully completed a training program approved by the Secretary and

(ii) homemaker services,

(E) medical supplies (including drugs and biologicals) and the use of medical appliances, while under such a plan,

(F) physicians' services,

(G) short-term inpatient care (including both respite care and procedures necessary for pain control and acute and chronic symptom management) in an inpatient facility meeting such conditions as the Secretary determines to be appropriate to provide such care, but such respite care may be provided only on an intermittent, nonroutine, and occasional basis and may not be provided consecutively over longer than five days,

(H) counseling (including dietary counseling) with respect to care of the terminally ill individual and adjustment to his death, and

(I) any other item or service which is specified in the plan and for which payment may otherwise be made under this title.

The care and services described in subparagraphs (A) and (D) may be provided on a 24-hour, continuous basis only during periods of crisis (meeting criteria established by the Secretary) and only as necessary to maintain the terminally ill individual at home.

(2) The term “hospice program” means a public agency or private organization (or a subdivision thereof) which—

(A)(i) is primarily engaged in providing the care and services described in paragraph (1) and makes such services available (as needed) on a 24-hour basis and which also provides bereavement counseling for the immediate family of terminally ill individuals and services described in section 1812(a)(5),

(ii) provides for such care and services in individuals’ homes, on an outpatient basis, and on a short-term inpatient basis, directly or under arrangements made by the agency or organization, except that—

(I) the agency or organization must routinely provide directly substantially all of each of the services described in subparagraphs (A), (C), and (H) of paragraph (1), except as otherwise provided in paragraph (5), and

(II) in the case of other services described in paragraph

(1) which are not provided directly by the agency or organization, the agency or organization must maintain professional management responsibility for all such services furnished to an individual, regardless of the location or facility in which such services are furnished; and

(iii) provides assurances satisfactory to the Secretary that the aggregate number of days of inpatient care described in paragraph (1)(G) provided in any 12-month period to individuals who have an election in effect under section 1812(d) with respect to that agency or organization does not exceed 20 percent of the aggregate number of days during that period on which such elections for such individuals are in effect;

(B) has an interdisciplinary group of personnel which—

(i) includes at least—

(I) one physician (as defined in subsection (r)(1)),

(II) one registered professional nurse, and

(III) one social worker,

employed by or, in the case of a physician described in sub-clause (I), under contract with the agency or organization, and also includes at least one pastoral or other counselor,

(ii) provides (or supervises the provision of) the care and services described in paragraph (1), and

(iii) establishes the policies governing the provision of such care and services;

(C) maintains central clinical records on all patients;

(D) does not discontinue the hospice care it provides with respect to a patient because of the inability of the patient to pay for such care;

(E)(i) utilizes volunteers in its provision of care and services in accordance with standards set by the Secretary, which standards shall ensure a continuing level of effort to utilize such volunteers, and (ii) maintains records on the use of these volunteers and the cost savings and expansion of care and services achieved through the use of these volunteers;

(F) in the case of an agency or organization in any State in which State or applicable local law provides for the licensing of agencies or organizations of this nature, is licensed pursuant to such law; and

(G) meets such other requirements as the Secretary may find necessary in the interest of the health and safety of the individuals who are provided care and services by such agency or organization.

(3)(A) An individual is considered to be "terminally ill" if the individual has a medical prognosis that the individual's life expectancy is 6 months or less.

(B) The term "attending physician" means, with respect to an individual, the physician (as defined in subsection (r)(1)), the nurse practitioner (as defined in subsection (aa)(5)), or the physician assistant (as defined in such subsection), who may be employed by a hospice program, whom the individual identifies as having the most significant role in the determination and delivery of medical care to the individual at the time the individual makes an election to receive hospice care.

(4)(A) An entity which is certified as a provider of services other than a hospice program shall be considered, for purposes of certification as a hospice program, to have met any requirements under paragraph (2) which are also the same requirements for certification as such other type of provider. The Secretary shall coordinate surveys for determining certification under this title so as to provide, to the extent feasible, for simultaneous surveys of an entity which seeks to be certified as a hospice program and as a provider of services of another type.

(B) Any entity which is certified as a hospice program and as a provider of another type shall have separate provider agreements under section 1866 and shall file separate cost reports with respect to costs incurred in providing hospice care and in providing other services and items under this title.

(C) Any entity that is certified as a hospice program shall be subject to a standard survey by an appropriate State or local survey agency, or an approved accreditation agency, as determined by the Secretary, not less frequently than once every 36 months beginning 6 months after the date of the enactment of this subparagraph and ending September 30, 2025.

(5)(A) The Secretary may waive the requirements of paragraph (2)(A)(ii)(I) for an agency or organization with respect to all or part of the nursing care described in paragraph (1)(A) if such agency or organization—

(i) is located in an area which is not an urbanized area (as defined by the Bureau of the Census);

(ii) was in operation on or before January 1, 1983; and

(iii) has demonstrated a good faith effort (as determined by the Secretary) to hire a sufficient number of nurses to provide such nursing care directly.

(B) Any waiver, which is in such form and containing such information as the Secretary may require and which is requested by an agency or organization under subparagraph (A) or (C), shall be deemed to be granted unless such request is denied by the Secretary within 60 days after the date such request is received by the Secretary. The granting of a waiver under subparagraph (A) or (C) shall not preclude the granting of any subsequent waiver request should such a waiver again become necessary.

(C) The Secretary may waive the requirements of paragraph (2)(A)(i) and (2)(A)(ii) for an agency or organization with respect to the services described in paragraph (1)(B) and, with respect to dietary counseling, paragraph (1)(H), if such agency or organization—

(i) is located in an area which is not an urbanized area (as defined by the Bureau of Census), and

(ii) demonstrates to the satisfaction of the Secretary that the agency or organization has been unable, despite diligent efforts, to recruit appropriate personnel.

(D) In extraordinary, exigent, or other non-routine circumstances, such as unanticipated periods of high patient loads, staffing shortages due to illness or other events, or temporary travel of a patient outside a hospice program's service area, a hospice program may enter into arrangements with another hospice program for the provision by that other program of services described in paragraph (2)(A)(ii)(I). The provisions of paragraph (2)(A)(ii)(II) shall apply with respect to the services provided under such arrangements.

(E) A hospice program may provide services described in paragraph (1)(A) other than directly by the program if the services are highly specialized services of a registered professional nurse and are provided non-routinely and so infrequently so that the provision of such services directly would be impracticable and prohibitively expensive.

### *Discharge Planning Process*

(ee)(1) A discharge planning process of a hospital shall be considered sufficient if it is applicable to services furnished by the hospital to individuals entitled to benefits under this title and if it meets the guidelines and standards established by the Secretary under paragraph (2).

(2) The Secretary shall develop guidelines and standards for the discharge planning process in order to ensure a timely and smooth transition to the most appropriate type of and setting for post-hospital or rehabilitative care. The guidelines and standards shall include the following:

(A) The hospital must identify, at an early stage of hospitalization, those patients who are likely to suffer adverse health consequences upon discharge in the absence of adequate discharge planning.

(B) Hospitals must provide a discharge planning evaluation for patients identified under subparagraph (A) and for other patients upon the request of the patient, patient's representative, or patient's physician.

(C) Any discharge planning evaluation must be made on a timely basis to ensure that appropriate arrangements for post-hospital care will be made before discharge and to avoid unnecessary delays in discharge.

(D) A discharge planning evaluation must include an evaluation of a patient's likely need for appropriate post-hospital services, including hospice care and post-hospital extended care services, and the availability of those services, including the availability of home health services through individuals and entities that participate in the program under this title and that serve the area in which the patient resides and that request to be listed by the hospital as available and, in the case of individuals who are likely to need post-hospital extended care services, the availability of such services through facilities that participate in the program under this title and that serve the area in which the patient resides.

(E) The discharge planning evaluation must be included in the patient's medical record for use in establishing an appropriate discharge plan and the results of the evaluation must be discussed with the patient (or the patient's representative).

(F) Upon the request of a patient's physician, the hospital must arrange for the development and initial implementation of a discharge plan for the patient.

(G) Any discharge planning evaluation or discharge plan required under this paragraph must be developed by, or under the supervision of, a registered professional nurse, social worker, or other appropriately qualified personnel.

(H) Consistent with section 1802, the discharge plan shall—

(i) not specify or otherwise limit the qualified provider which may provide post-hospital home health services, and

(ii) identify (in a form and manner specified by the Secretary) any entity to whom the individual is referred in which the hospital has a disclosable financial interest (as specified by the Secretary consistent with section 1866(a)(1)(S)) or which has such an interest in the hospital.

(3) With respect to a discharge plan for an individual who is enrolled with a Medicare+Choice organization under a Medicare+Choice plan and is furnished inpatient hospital services by a hospital under a contract with the organization—

(A) the discharge planning evaluation under paragraph (2)(D) is not required to include information on the availability of home health services through individuals and entities which do not have a contract with the organization; and

(B) notwithstanding subparagraph (H)(i), the plan may specify or limit the provider (or providers) of post-hospital home health services or other post-hospital services under the plan.

***Partial Hospitalization Services***

(ff)(1) The term "partial hospitalization services" means the items and services described in paragraph (2) prescribed by a physician and provided under a program described in paragraph (3) under the supervision of a physician pursuant to an individualized, written plan of treatment established and periodically reviewed by a physician (in consultation with appropriate staff participating in such program), which plan sets forth the physician's diagnosis, the type, amount, frequency, and duration of the items and services provided under the plan, and the goals for treatment under the plan.

(2) The items and services described in this paragraph are—

(A) individual and group therapy with physicians or psychologists (or other mental health professionals to the extent authorized under State law),

(B) occupational therapy requiring the skills of a qualified occupational therapist,

(C) services of social workers, trained psychiatric nurses, and other staff trained to work with psychiatric patients,

(D) drugs and biologicals furnished for therapeutic purposes (which cannot, as determined in accordance with regulations, be self-administered),

(E) individualized activity therapies that are not primarily recreational or diversionary,

(F) family counseling (the primary purpose of which is treatment of the individual's condition),

(G) patient training and education (to the extent that training and educational activities are closely and clearly related to individual's care and treatment),

(H) diagnostic services, and

(I) such other items and services as the Secretary may provide (but in no event to include meals and transportation);

that are reasonable and necessary for the diagnosis or active treatment of the individual's condition, reasonably expected to improve or maintain the individual's condition and functional level and to prevent relapse or hospitalization, and furnished pursuant to such guidelines relating to frequency and duration of services as the Secretary shall by regulation establish (taking into account accepted norms of medical practice and the reasonable expectation of patient improvement).

(3)(A) A program described in this paragraph is a program which is furnished by a hospital to its outpatients or by a community mental health center (as defined in subparagraph (B)), and which is a distinct and organized intensive ambulatory treatment service offering less than 24-hour-daily care other than in an individual's home or in an inpatient or residential setting.

(B) For purposes of subparagraph (A), the term "community mental health center" means an entity that—

(i)(I) provides the mental health services described in section 1913(c)(1) of the Public Health Service Act; or

(II) in the case of an entity operating in a State that by law precludes the entity from providing itself the service described in subparagraph (E) of such section, provides for such service by contract with an approved organization or entity (as determined by the Secretary);

(ii) meets applicable licensing or certification requirements for community mental health centers in the State in which it is located;

(iii) provides at least 40 percent of its services to individuals who are not eligible for benefits under this title; and

(iv) meets such additional conditions as the Secretary shall specify to ensure (I) the health and safety of individuals being furnished such services, (II) the effective and efficient furnishing of such services, and (III) the compliance of such entity with the criteria described in section 1931(c)(1) of the Public Health Service Act.

### *Certified Nurse-Midwife Services*

(gg)(1) The term "certified nurse-midwife services" means such services furnished by a certified nurse-midwife (as defined in paragraph (2)) and such services and supplies furnished as an incident to the nurse-midwife's service which the certified nurse-midwife is legally authorized to perform under State law (or the State regulatory mechanism provided by State law) as would otherwise be covered if furnished by a physician or as an incident to a physicians' service.

(2) The term "certified nurse-midwife" means a registered nurse who has successfully completed a program of study and clinical experience meeting guidelines prescribed by the Secretary, or has been certified by an organization recognized by the Secretary.

### *Clinical Social Worker; Clinical Social Worker Services*

(hh)(1) The term "clinical social worker" means an individual who—

(A) possesses a master's or doctor's degree in social work;

(B) after obtaining such degree has performed at least 2 years of supervised clinical social work; and

(C)(i) is licensed or certified as a clinical social worker by the State in which the services are performed, or

(ii) in the case of an individual in a State which does not provide for licensure or certification—

(I) has completed at least 2 years or 3,000 hours of postmaster's degree supervised clinical social work practice under the supervision of a master's level social worker in an appropriate setting (as determined by the Secretary), and

(II) meets such other criteria as the Secretary establishes.

(2) The term "clinical social worker services" means services performed by a clinical social worker (as defined in paragraph (1)) for the diagnosis and treatment of mental illnesses (other than services furnished to an inpatient of a hospital and other than services furnished to an inpatient of a skilled nursing facility which the facility is required to provide as a requirement for participation) which the clinical social worker is legally authorized to perform under State law (or the State regulatory mechanism provided by State law) of the State in which such services are performed as would otherwise be covered if furnished by a physician or as an incident to a physician's professional service.

### *Qualified Psychologist Services*

(ii) The term "qualified psychologist services" means such services and such services and supplies furnished as an incident to his service furnished by a clinical psychologist (as defined by the Secretary) which the psychologist is legally authorized to perform under State law (or the State regulatory mechanism provided by State law) as would otherwise be covered if furnished by a physician or as an incident to a physician's service.

### *Screening Mammography*

(jj) The term "screening mammography" means a radiologic procedure provided to a woman for the purpose of early detection of breast cancer and includes a physician's interpretation of the results of the procedure.

### *Covered Osteoporosis Drug*

(kk) The term "covered osteoporosis drug" means an injectable drug approved for the treatment of post-menopausal osteoporosis provided to an individual by a home health agency if, in accordance with regulations promulgated by the Secretary—

(1) the individual's attending physician certifies that the individual has suffered a bone fracture related to post-menopausal osteoporosis and that the individual is unable to learn the skills needed to self-administer such

drug or is otherwise physically or mentally incapable of self-administering such drug; and

(2) the individual is confined to the individual's home (except when receiving items and services referred to in subsection (m)(7)).

***Speech-Language Pathology Services; Audiology Services***

(ll)(1) The term "speech-language pathology services" means such speech, language, and related function assessment and rehabilitation services furnished by a qualified speech-language pathologist as the speech-language pathologist is legally authorized to perform under State law (or the State regulatory mechanism provided by State law) as would otherwise be covered if furnished by a physician.

(2) The term "outpatient speech-language pathology services" has the meaning given the term "outpatient physical therapy services" in subsection (p), except that in applying such subsection—

(A) "speech-language pathology" shall be substituted for "physical therapy" each place it appears; and

(B) "speech-language pathologist" shall be substituted for "physical therapist" each place it appears.

(3) The term "audiology services" means such hearing and balance assessment services furnished by a qualified audiologist as the audiologist is legally authorized to perform under State law (or the State regulatory mechanism provided by State law), as would otherwise be covered if furnished by a physician.

(4) In this subsection:

(A) The term "qualified speech-language pathologist" means an individual with a master's or doctoral degree in speech-language pathology who—

(i) is licensed as a speech-language pathologist by the State in which the individual furnishes such services, or

(ii) in the case of an individual who furnishes services in a State which does not license speech-language pathologists, has successfully completed 350 clock hours of supervised clinical practicum (or is in the process of accumulating such supervised clinical experience), performed not less than

9 months of supervised full-time speech-language pathology services after obtaining a master's or doctoral degree in speech-language pathology or a related field, and successfully completed a national examination in speech-language pathology approved by the Secretary.

(B) The term "qualified audiologist" means an individual with a master's or doctoral degree in audiology who—

(i) is licensed as an audiologist by the State in which the individual furnishes such services, or

(ii) in the case of an individual who furnishes services in a State which does not license audiologists, has successfully completed 350 clock hours of supervised clinical practicum (or is in the process of accumulating such supervised clinical experience), performed not less than 9 months of supervised full-time audiology services after obtaining a master's or doctoral degree in audiology or a related field, and successfully completed a national examination in audiology approved by the Secretary.

Critical Access Hospital; Critical Access Hospital Services (mm)(1) The term "critical access hospital" means a facility certified by the Secretary as a critical access hospital under section 1820(e).

(2) The term "inpatient critical access hospital services" means items and services, furnished to an inpatient of a critical access hospital by such facility, that would be inpatient hospital services if furnished to an inpatient of a hospital by a hospital.

(3) The term "outpatient critical access hospital services" means medical and other health services furnished by a critical access hospital on an outpatient basis.

### *Screening Pap Smear; Screening Pelvic Exam*

(nn)(1) The term "screening pap smear" means a diagnostic laboratory test consisting of a routine exfoliative cytology test (Papanicolaou test) provided to a woman for the purpose of early detection of cervical or vaginal cancer and includes a physician's interpretation of the results of the test, if the individual involved has not had such a test during the preceding 2 years, or during the preceding year in the case of a woman described in paragraph (3).

(2) The term "screening pelvic exam" means a pelvic examination provided to a woman if the woman involved has not had such an examination during the preceding 2 years, or during the preceding year in the case of a woman described in paragraph (3), and includes a clinical breast examination.

(3) A woman described in this paragraph is a woman who—

(A) is of childbearing age and has had a test described in this subsection during any of the preceding 3 years that indicated the presence of cervical or vaginal cancer or other abnormality; or

(B) is at high risk of developing cervical or vaginal cancer (as determined pursuant to factors identified by the Secretary).

***Prostate Cancer Screening Tests***

(oo)(1) The term "prostate cancer screening test" means a test that consists of any (or all) of the procedures described in paragraph (2) provided for the purpose of early detection of prostate cancer to a man over 50 years of age who has not had such a test during the preceding year.

(2) The procedures described in this paragraph are as follows:

(A) A digital rectal examination.

(B) A prostate-specific antigen blood test.

(C) For years beginning after 2002, such other procedures as the Secretary finds appropriate for the purpose of early detection of prostate cancer, taking into account changes in technology and standards of medical practice, availability, effectiveness, costs, and such other factors as the Secretary considers appropriate.

***Colorectal Cancer Screening Tests***

(pp)(1) The term "colorectal cancer screening test" means any of the following procedures furnished to an individual for the purpose of early detection of colorectal cancer:

(A) Screening fecal-occult blood test.

(B) Screening flexible sigmoidoscopy.

(C) Screening colonoscopy.

(D) Such other tests or procedures, and modifications to tests and procedures under this subsection, with such frequency and payment limits, as the Secretary determines appropriate, in consultation with appropriate organizations.

(2) An "individual at high risk for colorectal cancer" is an individual who, because of family history, prior experience of cancer or precursor neoplastic polyps, a history of chronic digestive disease condition (including inflammatory bowel disease, Crohn's Disease, or ulcerative colitis), the presence of any appropriate recognized gene markers for colorectal cancer, or other predisposing factors, faces a high risk for colorectal cancer.

***Diabetes Outpatient Self-Management Training Services***

(qq)(1) The term "diabetes outpatient self-management training services" means educational and training services furnished (at such times as the Secretary determines appropriate) to an individual with diabetes by a certified provider (as described in paragraph (2)(A)) in an outpatient setting by an individual or entity who meets the quality standards described in paragraph (2)(B), but only if the physician who is managing the individual's diabetic condition certifies that such services are needed under a comprehensive plan of care related to the individual's diabetic condition to ensure therapy compliance or to provide the individual with necessary skills and knowledge (including skills related to the self-administration of injectable drugs) to participate in the management of the individual's condition.

(2) In paragraph (1)—

(A) a "certified provider" is a physician, or other individual or entity designated by the Secretary, that, in addition to providing diabetes outpatient self-management training services, provides other items or services for which payment may be made under this title; and

(B) a physician, or such other individual or entity, meets the quality standards described in this paragraph if the physician, or individual or entity, meets quality standards established by the Secretary, except that the physician or other individual or entity shall be deemed to have met such standards if the physician or other individual or entity meets applicable standards originally established by the National Diabetes Advisory Board and subsequently revised by organizations who participated in the establishment of standards by such Board, or is recognized by an organization that represents individuals (including individuals under this title) with diabetes as meeting standards for furnishing the services.

### *Bone Mass Measurement*

(rr)(1) The term "bone mass measurement" means a radiologic or radioisotopic procedure or other procedure approved by the Food and Drug Administration performed on a qualified individual (as defined in paragraph (2)) for the purpose of identifying bone mass or detecting bone loss or determining bone quality, and includes a physician's interpretation of the results of the procedure.

(2) For purposes of this subsection, the term "qualified individual" means an individual who is (in accordance with regulations prescribed by the Secretary)—

(A) an estrogen-deficient woman at clinical risk for osteoporosis;

(B) an individual with vertebral abnormalities;

(C) an individual receiving long-term glucocorticoid steroid therapy;

(D) an individual with primary hyperparathyroidism; or

(E) an individual being monitored to assess the response to or efficacy of an approved osteoporosis drug therapy.

(3) The Secretary shall establish such standards regarding the frequency with which a qualified individual shall be eligible to be provided benefits for bone mass measurement under this title.

### *Religious Nonmedical Health Care Institution*

(ss)(1) The term "religious nonmedical health care institution" means an institution that—

(A) is described in subsection (c)(3) of section 501 of the Internal Revenue Code of 1986 and is exempt from taxes under subsection (a) of such section;

(B) is lawfully operated under all applicable Federal, State, and local laws and regulations;

(C) provides only nonmedical nursing items and services exclusively to patients who choose to rely solely upon a religious method of healing and for whom the acceptance of medical health services would be inconsistent with their religious beliefs;

(D) provides such nonmedical items and services exclusively through nonmedical nursing personnel who are experienced in caring for the physical needs of such patients;

(E) provides such nonmedical items and services to inpatients on a 24-hour basis;

(F) on the basis of its religious beliefs, does not provide through its personnel or otherwise medical items and services (including any medical screening, examination, diagnosis, prognosis, treatment, or the administration of drugs) for its patients;

(G)(i) is not owned by, under common ownership with, or has an ownership interest in, a provider of medical treatment or services;

(ii) is not affiliated with—

(I) a provider of medical treatment or services, or

(II) an individual who has an ownership interest in a provider of medical treatment or services;

(H) has in effect a utilization review plan which—

(i) provides for the review of admissions to the institution, of the duration of stays therein, of cases of continuous extended duration, and of the items and services furnished by the institution,

(ii) requires that such reviews be made by an appropriate committee of the institution that includes the individuals responsible for overall administration and for supervision of nursing personnel at the institution,

(iii) provides that records be maintained of the meetings, decisions, and actions of such committee, and

(iv) meets such other requirements as the Secretary finds necessary to establish an effective utilization review plan;

(I) provides the Secretary with such information as the Secretary may require to implement section 1821, including information relating to quality of care and coverage determinations; and

(J) meets such other requirements as the Secretary finds necessary in the interest of the health and safety of individuals who are furnished services in the institution.

(2) To the extent that the Secretary finds that the accreditation of an institution by a State, regional, or national agency or association provides reasonable assurances that any or all of the requirements of paragraph (1) are met or exceeded, the Secretary may treat such institution as meeting the condition or conditions with respect to which the Secretary made such finding.

(3)(A)(i) In administering this subsection and section 1821, the Secretary shall not require any patient of a religious nonmedical health care institution to undergo medical screening, examination, diagnosis, prognosis, or treatment or to accept any other medical health care service, if such patient (or legal representative of the patient) objects thereto on religious grounds.

(ii) Clause (i) shall not be construed as preventing the Secretary from requiring under section 1821(a)(2) the provision of sufficient information regarding an individual's condition as a condition for receipt of benefits under part A for services provided in such an institution.

(B)(i) In administering this subsection and section 1821, the Secretary shall not subject a religious nonmedical health care institution or its personnel to any medical supervision, regulation, or control, insofar as such supervision, regulation, or control would be contrary to the religious beliefs observed by the institution or such personnel.

(ii) Clause (i) shall not be construed as preventing the Secretary from reviewing items and services billed by the institution to the extent the Secretary determines such review to be necessary to determine whether such items and services were not covered under part A, are excessive, or are fraudulent.

(4)(A) For purposes of paragraph (1)(G)(i), an ownership interest of less than 5 percent shall not be taken into account.

(B) For purposes of paragraph (1)(G)(ii), none of the following shall be considered to create an affiliation:

(i) An individual serving as an uncompensated director, trustee, officer, or other member of the governing body of a religious nonmedical health care institution.

(ii) An individual who is a director, trustee, officer, employee, or staff member of a religious nonmedical health care institution having a family relationship with an individual who is affiliated with (or has an ownership interest in) a provider of medical treatment or services.

(iii) An individual or entity furnishing goods or services as a vendor to both providers of medical treatment or services and religious nonmedical health care institutions.

***Post-Institutional Home Health Services; Home Health Spell of Illness***

(tt)(1) The term "post-institutional home health services" means home health services furnished to an individual—

(A) after discharge from a hospital or critical access hospital in which the individual was an inpatient for not less than 3 consecutive days before such discharge if such home health services were initiated within 14 days after the date of such discharge; or

(B) after discharge from a skilled nursing facility in which the individual was provided post-hospital extended care services if such home health services were initiated within 14 days after the date of such discharge.

(2) The term "home health spell of illness" with respect to any individual means a period of consecutive days—

(A) beginning with the first day (not included in a previous home health spell of illness) (i) on which such individual is furnished post-institutional home health services, and (ii) which occurs in a month for which the individual is entitled to benefits under part A, and

(B) ending with the close of the first period of 60 consecutive days thereafter on each of which the individual is neither an inpatient of a hospital or critical access hospital nor an inpatient of a facility described in section 1819(a)(1) or subsection (y)(1) nor provided home health services.

### *Screening for Glaucoma*

(uu) The term "screening for glaucoma" means a dilated eye examination with an intraocular pressure measurement, and a direct ophthalmoscopy or a slit-lamp biomicroscopic examination for the early detection of glaucoma which is furnished by or under the direct supervision of an optometrist or ophthalmologist who is legally authorized to furnish such services under State law (or the State regulatory mechanism provided by State law) of the State in which the services are furnished, as would otherwise be covered if furnished by a physician or as an incident to a physician's professional service, if the individual involved has not had such an examination in the preceding year.

### *Medical Nutrition Therapy Services; Registered Dietitian or Nutrition Professional*

(vv)(1) The term "medical nutrition therapy services" means nutritional diagnostic, therapy, and counseling services for the purpose of disease management which are furnished by a registered dietitian or nutrition professional (as defined in paragraph (2)) pursuant to a referral by a physician (as defined in subsection (r)(1)).

(2) Subject to paragraph (3), the term "registered dietitian or nutrition professional" means an individual who—

(A) holds a baccalaureate or higher degree granted by a regionally accredited college or university in the United States (or an equivalent foreign degree) with completion of the academic requirements of a program in nutrition or dietetics, as accredited by an appropriate national accreditation organization recognized by the Secretary for this purpose;

(B) has completed at least 900 hours of supervised dietetics practice under the supervision of a registered dietitian or nutrition professional; and

(C)(i) is licensed or certified as a dietitian or nutrition professional by the State in which the services are performed; or

(ii) in the case of an individual in a State that does not provide for such licensure or certification, meets such other criteria as the Secretary establishes.

(3) Subparagraphs (A) and (B) of paragraph (2) shall not apply in the case of an individual who, as of the date of the enactment of this subsection, is licensed or certified as a dietitian or nutrition professional by the State in which medical nutrition therapy services are performed.

***Initial Preventive Physical Examination***

(ww)(1) The term "initial preventive physical examination" means physicians' services consisting of a physical examination (including measurement of height, weight body mass index,, and blood pressure) with the goal of health promotion and disease detection and includes education, counseling, and referral with respect to screening and other preventive services described in paragraph (2) and end-of-life planning (as defined in paragraph (3)) upon the agreement with the individual, *and a review of current opioid prescriptions and screening for opioid use disorder (as defined in paragraph (4)),* but does not include clinical laboratory tests.

(2) The screening and other preventive services described in this paragraph include the following:

(A) Pneumococcal, influenza, and hepatitis B vaccine and administration under subsection (s)(10).

(B) Screening mammography as defined in subsection (jj).

(C) Screening pap smear and screening pelvic exam as defined in subsection (nn).

(D) Prostate cancer screening tests as defined in subsection (oo).

(E) Colorectal cancer screening tests as defined in subsection (pp).

(F) Diabetes outpatient self-management training services as defined in subsection (qq)(1).

(G) Bone mass measurement as defined in subsection (rr).

(H) Screening for glaucoma as defined in subsection (uu).

(I) Medical nutrition therapy services as defined in sub-section (vv).

(J) Cardiovascular screening blood tests as defined in subsection (xx)(1).

(K) Diabetes screening tests as defined in subsection (yy).

(L) Ultrasound screening for abdominal aortic aneurysm as defined in section 1861(bbb).

(M) An electrocardiogram.

(N) Additional preventive services (as defined in subsection (ddd)(1)).

(3) For purposes of paragraph (1), the term "end-of-life planning" means verbal or written information regarding—

(A) an individual's ability to prepare an advance directive in the case that an injury or illness causes the individual to be unable to make health care decisions; and

(B) whether or not the physician is willing to follow the individual's wishes as expressed in an advance directive.

(4)(A) For purposes of paragraph (1), the term "a review of current opioid prescriptions and screening for opioid use disorder" means, with respect to an individual—

(i) a review by a physician or qualified non-physician practitioner of all current prescriptions of the individual; and

(ii) in the case of an individual determined by the review of a physician or qualified non-physician practitioner under sub-paragraph (A) to have a current prescription for opioids for chronic pain that has been prescribed for a minimum period of time (as specified by the Secretary)—

(I) a review by the physician or practitioner of the potential risk factors to the individual for opioid use disorder;

(II) an evaluation by the physician or practitioner of pain of the individual;

(III) the provision of information regarding non-opioid treatment options for the treatment and management of any chronic pain of the individual; and

(IV) if determined necessary by the physician or practitioner based on the results of the review and evaluation conducted as described in this paragraph, an appropriate referral by the physician or practitioner for additional treatment.

(B) For purposes of this paragraph, the term "qualified non-physician practitioner" means a physician assistant, nurse practitioner, or certified clinical nurse specialist.

### *Cardiovascular Screening Blood Test*

(xx)(1) The term "cardiovascular screening blood test" means a blood test for the early detection of cardiovascular disease (or abnormalities associated with an elevated risk of cardiovascular disease) that tests for the following:

(A) Cholesterol levels and other lipid or triglyceride levels.

(B) Such other indications associated with the presence of, or an elevated risk for, cardiovascular disease as the Secretary may approve for all individuals (or for some individuals determined by the Secretary to be at risk for cardiovascular disease), including indications measured by noninvasive testing.

The Secretary may not approve an indication under subparagraph

(B) for any individual unless a blood test for such is recommended by the United States Preventive Services Task Force.

(2) The Secretary shall establish standards, in consultation with appropriate organizations, regarding the frequency for each type of cardiovascular screening blood tests, except that such frequency may not be more often than once every 2 years.

### *Diabetes Screening Tests*

(yy)(1) The term "diabetes screening tests" means testing furnished to an individual at risk for diabetes (as defined in paragraph (2)) for the purpose of early detection of diabetes, including—

(A) a fasting plasma glucose test; and

(B) such other tests, and modifications to tests, as the Secretary determines appropriate, in consultation with appropriate organizations.

(2) For purposes of paragraph (1), the term "individual at risk for diabetes" means an individual who has any of the following risk factors for diabetes:

(A) Hypertension.

(B) Dyslipidemia.

(C) Obesity, defined as a body mass index greater than or equal to 30 kg/m2.

(D) Previous identification of an elevated impaired fasting glucose.

(E) Previous identification of impaired glucose tolerance.

(F) A risk factor consisting of at least 2 of the following characteristics:

(i) Overweight, defined as a body mass index greater than 25, but less than 30, kg/m2.

(ii) A family history of diabetes.

(iii) A history of gestational diabetes mellitus or delivery of a baby weighing greater than 9 pounds.

(iv) 65 years of age or older.

(3) The Secretary shall establish standards, in consultation with appropriate organizations, regarding the frequency of diabetes screening tests, except that such frequency may not be more often than twice within the 12-month period following the date of the most recent diabetes screening test of that individual.

### *Intravenous Immune Globulin*

(zz) The term "intravenous immune globulin" means an approved pooled plasma derivative for the treatment in the patient's home of a patient with a diagnosed primary immune deficiency disease, but not including items or services related to the administration of the derivative, if a physician determines administration of the derivative in the patient's home is medically appropriate.

### *Extended Care in Religious Nonmedical Health Care Institutions*

(aaa)(1) The term "home health agency" also includes a religious nonmedical health care institution (as defined in subsection (ss)(1)), but only with respect to items and services ordinarily furnished by such an institution to individuals in their homes, and that are comparable to items and services furnished to individuals by a home health agency that is not religious nonmedical health care institution.

(2)(A) Subject to subparagraphs (B), payment may be made with respect to services provided by such an institution only to such extent and under such conditions, limitations, and requirements (in addition to or in lieu of the conditions, limitations, and requirements otherwise applicable) as may be provided in regulations consistent with section 1821.

(B) Notwithstanding any other provision of this title, payment may not be made under subparagraph (A)—

(i) in a year insofar as such payments exceed $700,000; and

(ii) after December 31, 2006.

***Ultrasound Screening for Abdominal Aortic Aneurysm***

(bbb) The term "ultrasound screening for abdominal aortic aneurysm" means—

(1) a procedure using sound waves (or such other procedures using alternative technologies, of commensurate accuracy and cost, that the Secretary may specify) provided for the early detection of abdominal aortic aneurysm; and

(2) includes a physician's interpretation of the results of the procedure.

***Long-Term Care Hospital***

(ccc) The term "long-term care hospital" means a hospital which—

(1) is primarily engaged in providing inpatient services, by or under the supervision of a physician, to Medicare beneficiaries whose medically complex conditions require a long hospital stay and programs of care provided by a long-term care hospital;

(2) has an average inpatient length of stay (as determined by the Secretary) of greater than 25 days, or meets the requirements of clause (II) of section 1886(d)(1)(B)(iv);

(3) satisfies the requirements of subsection (e); and

(4) meets the following facility criteria:

(A) the institution has a patient review process, documented in the patient medical record, that screens patients prior to admission for appropriateness of admission to a long-term care hospital, validates within 48 hours of admission that patients meet admission criteria for long-term care hospitals, regularly evaluates patients through- out their stay for continuation of care in a long-term care hospital, and assesses the available discharge options when patients no longer meet such continued stay criteria;

(B) the institution has active physician involvement with patients during their treatment through an organized medical staff, physician-directed treatment with physician on-site availability on a daily basis to review patient progress, and consulting physicians on call and capable of being at the patient's side within a moderate period of time, as determined by the Secretary; and

(C) the institution has interdisciplinary team treatment for patients, requiring interdisciplinary teams of health care professionals, including physicians, to prepare and carry out an individualized treatment plan for each patient.

***Additional Preventive Services; Preventive Services***

(ddd)(1) The term "additional preventive services" means services not described in subparagraph (A) or (C) of paragraph (3) that identify medical conditions or risk factors and that the Secretary determines are—

(A) reasonable and necessary for the prevention or early detection of an illness or disability;

(B) recommended with a grade of A or B by the United States Preventive Services Task Force; and

(C) appropriate for individuals entitled to benefits under part A or enrolled under part B.

(2) In making determinations under paragraph (1) regarding the coverage of a new service, the Secretary shall use the process for making national coverage determinations (as defined in section 1869(f)(1)(B)) under this title. As part of the use of such process, the Secretary may conduct an assessment of the relation between predicted outcomes and the expenditures for such service and may take into account the results of such assessment in making such determination.

(3) The term "preventive services" means the following:

(A) The screening and preventive services described in subsection (ww)(2) (other than the service described in subparagraph (M) of such subsection).

(B) An initial preventive physical examination (as defined in subsection (ww)).

(C) Personalized prevention plan services (as defined in subsection (hhh)(1)).

Cardiac Rehabilitation Program; Intensive Cardiac Rehabilitation Program

(eee)(1) The term "cardiac rehabilitation program" means a program (as described in paragraph (2)) that furnishes the items and services described in paragraph (3) under the supervision of a physician (as defined in subsection (r)(1)) or a physician assistant, nurse practitioner, or clinical nurse specialist (as those terms are defined in subsection (aa)(5)).

(2) A program described in this paragraph is a program under which—

(A) items and services under the program are delivered—

(i) in a physician's office;

(ii) in a hospital on an outpatient basis; or

(iii) in other settings determined appropriate by the Secretary;

(B) a physician (as defined in subsection (r)(1)) or a physician assistant, nurse practitioner, or clinical nurse specialist (as those terms are defined in subsection (aa)(5)) is immediately available and accessible for medical consultation and medical emergencies at all times items and services are being furnished under the program, except that, in the case of items and services furnished under such a program in a hospital, such availability shall be presumed; and

(C) individualized treatment is furnished under a written plan established, reviewed, and signed by a physician every 30 days that describes—

(i) the individual's diagnosis;

(ii) the type, amount, frequency, and duration of the items and services furnished under the plan; and

(iii) the goals set for the individual under the plan.

(3) The items and services described in this paragraph are—

(A) physician-prescribed exercise;

(B) cardiac risk factor modification, including education, counseling, and behavioral intervention (to the extent such education, counseling, and behavioral intervention is closely related to the individual's care and treatment and is tailored to the individual's needs);

(C) psychosocial assessment;

(D) outcomes assessment; and

(E) such other items and services as the Secretary may determine, but only if such items and services are—

(i) reasonable and necessary for the diagnosis or active treatment of the individual's condition;

(ii) reasonably expected to improve or maintain the individual's condition and functional level; and

(iii) furnished under such guidelines relating to the frequency and duration of such items and services as the Secretary shall establish, taking into account accepted norms of medical practice and the reasonable expectation of improvement of the individual.

(4)(A) The term "intensive cardiac rehabilitation program" means a program (as described in paragraph (2)) that furnishes the items and services described in paragraph (3) under the supervision of a physician (as defined in subsection (r)(1)) or a physician assistant, nurse practitioner, or clinical nurse specialist (as those terms are defined in subsection (aa)(5)) and has shown, in peer-reviewed published research, that it accomplished—

(i) one or more of the following:

(I) positively affected the progression of coronary heart disease; or

(II) reduced the need for coronary bypass surgery; or

(III) reduced the need for percutaneous coronary interventions; and

(ii) a statistically significant reduction in 5 or more of the following measures from their level before receipt of cardiac rehabilitation services to their level after receipt of such services:

(I) low density lipoprotein;

(II) triglycerides;

(III) body mass index;

(IV) systolic blood pressure;

(V) diastolic blood pressure; or

(VI) the need for cholesterol, blood pressure, and diabetes medications.

(B) To be eligible for an intensive cardiac rehabilitation program, an individual must have—

(i) had an acute myocardial infarction within the preceding 12 months;

(ii) had coronary bypass surgery;

(iii) stable angina pectoris;

(iv) had heart valve repair or replacement;

(v) had percutaneous transluminal coronary angioplasty (PTCA) or coronary stenting;

(vi) had a heart or heart-lung transplant;

(vii) stable, chronic heart failure (defined as patients with left ventricular ejection fraction of 35 percent or less and New York Heart Association (NYHA) class II to IV symptoms despite being on optimal heart failure therapy for at least 6 weeks); or

(viii) any additional condition for which the Secretary has determined that a cardiac rehabilitation program shall be covered, unless the Secretary determines, using the same process used to determine that the condition is covered for a cardiac rehabilitation program, that such coverage is not supported by the clinical evidence.

(C) An intensive cardiac rehabilitation program may be provided in a series of 72 one-hour sessions (as defined in section 1848(b)(5)), up to 6 sessions per day, over a period of up to 18 weeks.

(5) The Secretary shall establish standards to ensure that a physician with expertise in the management of individuals with cardiac pathophysiology who is licensed to practice medicine in the State in which a cardiac rehabilitation program (or the intensive cardiac rehabilitation program, as the case may be) is offered—

(A) is responsible for such program; and

(B) in consultation with appropriate staff, is involved substantially in directing the progress of individual in the program.

***Pulmonary Rehabilitation Program***

(fff)(1) The term "pulmonary rehabilitation program" means a program (as described in subsection (eee)(2) with respect to a program under this subsection) that furnishes the items and services described in paragraph (2) under the supervision of a physician (as defined in subsection (r)(1)) or a physician assistant, nurse practitioner, or clinical nurse specialist (as those terms are defined in subsection (aa)(5)).

(2) The items and services described in this paragraph are—

(A) physician-prescribed exercise;

(B) education or training (to the extent the education or training is closely and clearly related to the individual's care and treatment and is tailored to such individual's needs);

(C) psychosocial assessment;

(D) outcomes assessment; and

(E) such other items and services as the Secretary may determine, but only if such items and services are—

(i) reasonable and necessary for the diagnosis or active treatment of the individual's condition;

(ii) reasonably expected to improve or maintain the individual's condition and functional level; and

(iii) furnished under such guidelines relating to the frequency and duration of such items and services as the Secretary shall establish, taking into account accepted norms of medical practice and the reasonable expectation of improvement of the individual.

(3) The Secretary shall establish standards to ensure that a physician with expertise in the management of individuals with respiratory pathophysiology who is licensed to practice medicine in the State in which a pulmonary rehabilitation program is offered—

(A) is responsible for such program; and

(B) in consultation with appropriate staff, is involved substantially in directing the progress of individual in the program.

***Kidney Disease Education Services***

(ggg)(1) The term "kidney disease education services" means educational services that are—

(A) furnished to an individual with stage IV chronic kidney disease who, according to accepted clinical guidelines identified by the Secretary, will require dialysis or a kidney transplant;

(B) furnished, upon the referral of the physician managing the individual's kidney condition, by a qualified person (as defined in paragraph (2)); and

(C) designed—

(i) to provide comprehensive information (consistent with the standards set under paragraph (3)) regarding—

(I) the management of comorbidities, including for purposes of delaying the need for dialysis;

(II) the prevention of uremic complications; and

(III) each option for renal replacement therapy (including hemodialysis and peritoneal dialysis at home and in-center as well as vascular access options and transplantation);

(ii) to ensure that the individual has the opportunity to actively participate in the choice of therapy; and

(iii) to be tailored to meet the needs of the individual involved.

(2)(A) The term "qualified person" means—

(i) a physician (as defined in section 1861(r)(1)) or a physician assistant, nurse practitioner, or clinical nurse specialist (as defined in section 1861(aa)(5)), who furnishes services for which payment may be made under the fee schedule established under section 1848; and

(ii) a provider of services located in a rural area (as defined in section 1886(d)(2)(D)).

(B) Such term does not include a provider of services (other than a provider of services described in subparagraph (A)(ii)) or a renal dialysis facility.

(3) The Secretary shall set standards for the content of such information to be provided under paragraph (1)(C)(i) after consulting with physicians, other health professionals, health educators, professional

organizations, accrediting organizations, kidney patient organizations, dialysis facilities, transplant centers, network organizations described in section 1881(c)(2), and other knowledgeable persons. To the extent possible the Secretary shall consult with persons or entities described in the previous sentence, other than a dialysis facility, that has not received industry funding from a drug or biological manufacturer or dialysis facility.

(4) No individual shall be furnished more than 6 sessions of kidney disease education services under this title.

***Annual Wellness Visit***

(hhh)(1) The term "personalized prevention plan services" means the creation of a plan for an individual—

(A) that includes a health risk assessment (that meets the guidelines established by the Secretary under paragraph (4)(A)) of the individual that is completed prior to or as part of the same visit with a health professional described in paragraph (3); and

(B) that—

(i) takes into account the results of the health risk assessment; and

(ii) may contain the elements described in paragraph (2).

(2) Subject to paragraph (4)(H), the elements described in this paragraph are the following:

(A) The establishment of, or an update to, the individual's medical and family history.

(B) A list of current providers and suppliers that are regularly involved in providing medical care to the individual (including a list of all prescribed medications).

(C) A measurement of height, weight, body mass index (or waist circumference, if appropriate), blood pressure, and other routine measurements.

(D) Detection of any cognitive impairment.

(E) The establishment of, or an update to, the following:

(i) A screening schedule for the next 5 to 10 years, as appropriate, based on recommendations of the United States Preventive Services Task

Force and the Advisory Committee on Immunization Practices, and the individual's health status, screening history, and age-appropriate preventive services covered under this title.

(ii) A list of risk factors and conditions for which primary, secondary, or tertiary prevention interventions are recommended or are underway, including any mental health conditions or any such risk factors or conditions that have been identified through an initial preventive physical examination (as described under subsection (ww)(1)), and a list of treatment options and their associated risks and benefits.

(F) The furnishing of personalized health advice and a referral, as appropriate, to health education or preventive counseling services or programs aimed at reducing identified risk factors and improving self-management, or community-based lifestyle interventions to reduce health risks and promote self-management and wellness, including weight loss, physical activity, smoking cessation, fall prevention, and nutrition.

(G) Any other element determined appropriate by the Secretary.

() A health professional described in this paragraph is—

(A) a physician;

(B) a practitioner described in clause (i) of section 1842(b)(18)(C); or

(C) a medical professional (including a health educator, registered dietitian, or nutrition professional) or a team of medical professionals, as determined appropriate by the Secretary, under the supervision of a physician.

(4)(A) For purposes of paragraph (1)(A), the Secretary, not later than 1 year after the date of enactment of this subsection, shall establish publicly available guidelines for health risk assessments. Such guidelines shall be developed in consultation with relevant groups and entities and shall provide that a health risk assessment—

(i) identify chronic diseases, injury risks, modifiable risk factors, and urgent health needs of the individual; and

(ii) may be furnished—

(I) through an interactive telephonic or web-based program that meets the standards established under subparagraph (B);

(II) during an encounter with a health care professional;

(III) through community-based prevention programs; or

(IV) through any other means the Secretary determines appropriate to maximize accessibility and ease of use by beneficiaries, while ensuring the privacy of such beneficiaries.

(B) Not later than 1 year after the date of enactment of this subsection, the Secretary shall establish standards for interactive telephonic or web-based programs used to furnish health risk assessments under subparagraph (A)(ii)(I). The Secretary may utilize any health risk assessment developed under section 4004(f) of the Patient Protection and Affordable Care Act as part of the requirement to develop a personalized prevention plan to comply with this sub-paragraph.

(C)(i) Not later than 18 months after the date of enactment of this subsection, the Secretary shall develop and make available to the public a health risk assessment model. Such model shall meet the guidelines under subparagraph (A) and may be used to meet the requirement under paragraph (1)(A).

(ii) Any health risk assessment that meets the guidelines under subparagraph (A) and is approved by the Secretary may be used to meet the requirement under paragraph (1)(A).

(D) The Secretary may coordinate with community-based entities (including State Health Insurance Programs, Area Agencies on Aging, Aging and Disability Resource Centers, and the Administration on Aging) to—

(i) ensure that health risk assessments are accessible to beneficiaries; and

(ii) provide appropriate support for the completion of health risk assessments by beneficiaries.

(E) The Secretary shall establish procedures to make beneficiaries and providers aware of the requirement that a beneficiary complete a health risk assessment prior to or at the same time as receiving personalized prevention plan services.

(F) To the extent practicable, the Secretary shall encourage the use of, integration with, and coordination of health information technology (including use of technology that is compatible with electronic medical records and personal health records) and may experiment with the use of personalized technology to aid in the development of self-management skills and management of and adherence to provider recommendations in order to improve the health status of beneficiaries.

(G) A beneficiary shall be eligible to receive only an initial preventive physical examination (as defined under subsection (ww)(1)) during the 12-month period after the date that the beneficiary's coverage begins under part B and shall be eligible to receive personalized prevention plan services under this subsection each year thereafter provided that the beneficiary has not received either an initial preventive physical examination or personalized prevention plan services within the preceding 12-month period.

(H) The Secretary shall issue guidance that—

(i) identifies elements under paragraph (2) that are required to be provided to a beneficiary as part of their first visit for personalized prevention plan services; and

(ii) establishes a yearly schedule for appropriate provision of such elements thereafter.

(iii) Home Infusion Therapy.—(1) The term "home infusion therapy" means the items and services described in paragraph (2) furnished by a qualified home infusion therapy supplier (as defined in paragraph (3)(D)) which are furnished in the individual's home (as defined in paragraph (3)(B)) to an individual—

(A) who is under the care of an applicable provider (as defined in paragraph (3)(A)); and

(B) with respect to whom a plan prescribing the type, amount, and duration of infusion therapy services that are to be furnished such individual has been established by a physician (as defined in subsection (r)(1)) and is periodically reviewed by a physician (as so defined) in coordination with the furnishing of home infusion drugs (as defined in paragraph (3)(C)) under part B.

(2) The items and services described in this paragraph are the following:

(A) Professional services, including nursing services, furnished in accordance with the plan.

(B) Training and education (not otherwise paid for as durable medical equipment (as defined in subsection (n)), remote monitoring, and monitoring services for the provision of home infusion therapy and home infusion drugs furnished by a qualified home infusion therapy supplier.

(3) For purposes of this subsection:

(A) The term "applicable provider" means—

(i) a physician;

(ii) a nurse practitioner; and

(iii) a physician assistant.

(B) The term "home" means a place of residence used as the home of an individual (as defined for purposes of subsection (n)).

(C) The term "home infusion drug" means a parenteral drug or biological administered intravenously, or subcutaneously for an administration period of 15 minutes or more, in the home of an individual through a pump that is an item of durable medical equipment (as defined in subsection (n)). Such term does not include the following:

(i) Insulin pump systems.

(ii) A self-administered drug or biological on a self-administered drug exclusion list.

(D)(i) The term "qualified home infusion therapy supplier" means a pharmacy, physician, or other provider of services or supplier licensed by the State in which the pharmacy, physician, or provider or services or supplier furnishes items or services and that—

(I) furnishes infusion therapy to individuals with acute or chronic conditions requiring administration of home infusion drugs;

(II) ensures the safe and effective provision and administration of home infusion therapy on a 7-day-a-week, 24-hour-a-day basis;

(III) is accredited by an organization designated by the Secretary pursuant to section 1834(u)(5); and

(IV) meets such other requirements as the Secretary determines appropriate, taking into account the standards of care for home infusion therapy established by Medicare Advantage plans under part C and in the private sector.

(ii) A qualified home infusion therapy supplier may sub-contract with a pharmacy, physician, provider of services, or supplier to meet the requirements of this subparagraph.

## Exchange of Letters with Additional Committees of Referral

One Hundred Fifteenth Congress
Congress of the United States
House of Representatives
Committee on Energy and Commerce
June 7, 2018

The Honorable Kevin Brady
Chairman
Committee on Ways and Means
II 02 Longworth House Office Building
Washington, DC 20515

Dear Chairman Brady:

On May 9 and 17, 2018, the Committee on Energy and Commerce ordered favorably reported over 50 bills to address the opioid epidemic facing communities across our nation. Several of the bills were also referred to the Committee on Ways and Means.

I ask that the Committee on Ways and Means not insist on its referral of the following bills so that they may be scheduled for consideration by the Majority Leader:

- H.R. 1925, At-Risk Youth Medicaid Protection Act of2017;
- H.R. 3331, To amend title XI of the Social Security Act to promote testing of incentive payments for behavioral health providers for adoption and use of certified electronic health record technology;
- H.R. 3528, Every Prescription Conveyed Securely Act;
- H.R.4841, Standardizing Electronic Prior Authorization for Safe Prescribing Act of 2018;
- H.R. 5582, Abuse Deterrent Access Act of2018;
- H.R. 5590, Opioid Addiction Action Plan Act;
- H.R. 5603, Access to Telehealth Services for Opioid Use Disorder;
- H.R. 5605, Advancing High Quality Treatment for Opioid Use Disorders in Medicare Act;
- H.R. 5675, To amend title XVIII of the Social Security Act to require prescription drug plan sponsors under the Medicare program to establish drug management programs for at-risk beneficiaries;
- H.R. 5684, Protecting Seniors from Opioid Abuse Act;
- H.R. 5685, Medicare Opioid Safety Education Act;
- H.R. 5686, Medicare Clear Health Options in Care for Enrollees (CHOICE) Act;
- H.R. 5715, Strengthening Partnerships to Prevent Opioid Abuse Act;
- H.R. 5716, Commit to Opioid Medical Prescriber Accountability and Safety for Seniors (COMPASS) Act;
- H.R. 5796, Responsible Education Achieves Care and Healthy Outcomes for Users' Treatment (REACH OUT) Act of2018;
- H.R. 5798, Opioid Screening and Chronic Pain Management Alternatives for Seniors Act;
- H.R. 5804, Post-Surgical injections as an Opioid Alternative Act; and
- H.R. 5809, Postoperative Opioid Prevention Act of2018.

This concession in no way affects your jurisdiction over the subject matter of these bills, and it will not serve as precedent for future referrals. In addition, should a conference on the bills be necessary, I would support your request to have the Committee on Ways and Means on the conference committee. Finally, I would be pleased to include this letter and your response in the bill reports and the Congressional Record.

Thank you for your consideration of my request and for the extraordinary cooperation shown by you and your staff over matters of shared jurisdiction. I look forward to further opportunities to work with you this Congress.

Sincerely,

The Honorable Greg Walden
Chairman
Congress of the United States
U.S. House of Representatives

Committee on Ways and Means
June 8, 2018
Committee on Energy and Commerce
2125 Rayburn House Office Building
Washington, DC 20515

Dear Chairman Walden,

Thank you for your letter concerning several bills favorably reported out of the Committee on Energy and Commerce to address the opioid epidemic and which the Committee on Ways and Means was granted an additional referral.

As a result of your having consulted with us on provisions within these bills that fall within the Rule X jurisdiction of the Committee on Ways and Means, I agree to waive formal consideration of the following bills so that they may move expeditiously to the floor:

- H.R.1925, At-Risk Youth Medicaid Protection Act of2017;
- H.R. 3331, To amend title XI of the Social Security Act to promote testing of incentive payments for behavioral health providers for adoption and use of certified electronic health record technology;
- H.R. 3528, Every Prescription Conveyed Securely Act;
- H.R. 4841, Standardizing Electronic Prior Authorization for Safe Prescribing Act of 2018;
- H.R.5582, Abuse Deterrent Access Act of2018;
- H.R. 5590, Opioid Addiction Action Plan Act;
- H.R. 5603, Access to Telehealth Services for Opioid Use Disorder;
- H.R. 5605, Advancing High Quality Treatment for Opioid Use Disorders in Medicare Act;
- H.R. 5675, To amend title XVIII of the Social Security Act to require prescription drug plan sponsors under the Medicare program to establish drug management programs for at-risk beneficiaries;
- H.R. 5684, Protecting Seniors from Opioid Abuse Act;
- H.R.5685, Medicare Opioid Safety Education Act;
- H.R.5686, Medicare Clear Health Options in Care for Enrollees (CHOICE) Act;
- H.R. 5715, Strengthening Partnerships to Prevent Opioid Abuse Act;
- H.R. 5716, Commit to Opioid Medical Prescriber Accountability and Safety for Seniors (COMPASS) Act;
- H.R. 5796, Responsible Education Achieves Care and Healthy Outcomes for Users' Treatment (REACH OUT) Act of2018;
- H.R.5798, Opioid Screening and Chronic Pain Management Alternatives for Seniors Act;
- H.R. 5804, Post-Surgical Injections as an Opioid Alternative Act; and
- H.R. 5809, Postoperative Opioid Prevention Act of 2018.

The Committee on Ways and Means takes this action with the mutual understanding that we do not waive any jurisdiction over the subject matter contained in this or similar legislation, and the Committee will be appropriately consulted and involved as the bill or similar legislation moves forward so that we may address any remaining issues that fall within our jurisdiction. The Committee also reserves the right to seek appointment of an appropriate number of conferees to any House-Senate conference involving this or similar legislation and requests your support for such a request.

Finally, I would appreciate your commitment to include this exchange of letters in the bill reports and the Congressional Record.

Sincerely,

Kevin Brady
Chairman

cc: The Honorable Paul Ryan, Speaker
The Honorable Richard E. Neal
The Honorable Frank Pallone
Thomas J. Wickham, Jr., Parliamentarian

In: Opioid Use and Misuse …
Editor: Tom Freitag
ISBN: 978-1-53616-858-7


*Chapter 2*

# ADVANCING HIGH QUALITY TREATMENT FOR OPIOID USE DISORDERS IN MEDICARE ACT*

*Committee on Energy and Commerce*

## PURPOSE AND SUMMARY

H.R. 5605, Advancing High Quality Treatment for Opioid Use Disorders in Medicare, was introduced on April 24, 2018, by Rep. Raul Ruiz (D–CA), to create a demonstration project to test new ways to treat opioid use disorder among the Medicare population. This model includes the development of measures to evaluate the quality and outcomes of treatment.

* This is an edited, reformatted and augmented version of House of Representatives Report, Committed to the Committee of the Whole House on the State of the Union and ordered to be printed, Publication No. 115–744, Part 1, dated June 12, 2018.

## Background and Need for Legislation

The Medicare program serves as the healthcare coverage provider to over 58 million beneficiaries. This number is projected to rise to over 80 million by 2030. In serving the over age 65 population, Medicare accounts for a large share of total opioid prescriptions. In 2016, one out of every three beneficiaries was prescribed an opioid through Medicare Part D. In total, this equates to almost 80 million prescriptions and $4 billion in Medicare Part D spending. While many Medicare beneficiaries with serious pain-related conditions are being properly prescribed opioids, there is mounting evidence of opioid misuse in the Medicare system. As more seniors and individuals with disabilities come into the program, the challenges of fraud, misuse, and abuse will only increase.

This bill seeks to increase beneficiary access to opioid use disorder treatment services, as well as improve physical and mental health outcomes for such beneficiaries through the creation of a new care based model. The bill would create an Alternative Payment Model (APM) demonstration program to incentivize the delivery of high quality, evidence-based substance use disorder treatment services, including both medication-assisted treatment as well as appropriate psychosocial supports. In conjunction with stakeholders, the Secretary would develop quality and outcome measures to assess the care beneficiaries receive through the Program. Participants would be eligible to receive incentive payment for providing quality substance use disorder treatment care.

## Committee Action

On April 11 and 12, 2018, the Subcommittee on Health held a hearing entitled "Combating the Opioid Crisis: Improving the Ability of Medicare and Medicaid to Provide Care for Patients" to review legislation related to the opioid epidemic. The Subcommittee received testimony from:

- Kimberly Brandt, Principal Deputy Administrator for Operations, Centers for Medicare and Medicaid Services, U.S. Department of Health and Human Services;
- Michael Botticelli, Executive Director, Grayken Center for Addiction, Boston Medical Center;
- Toby Douglas, Senior Vice President, Medicaid Solutions, Centene Corporation;
- David Guth, CEO, Centerstone;
- John Kravitz, CIO, Geisinger Health System; and,
- Sam Srivastava, CEO, Magellan Health.

On April 25, 2018, the Subcommittee on Health met in open markup session and forwarded a discussion draft, entitled "Alternative Payment Model for Treating Substance Use Disorder," without amendment, to the full Committee by a voice vote. On May 17, 2018, the full Committee on Energy and Commerce met in open markup session and ordered H.R. 5605, as amended, favorable reported to the House by a voice vote. H.R. 5605 was similar to the discussion draft forwarded by the Subcommittee.

## Committee Votes

Clause 3(b) of rule XIII requires the Committee to list the record votes on the motion to report legislation and amendments thereto. There were no record votes taken in connection with ordering H.R. 5605 reported.

## Oversight Findings and Recommendations

Pursuant to clause 2(b)(1) of rule X and clause 3(c)(1) of rule XIII, the Committee held a hearing and made findings that are reflected in this report.

## New Budget Authority, Entitlement Authority, and Tax Expenditures

Pursuant to clause 3(c)(2) of rule XIII, the Committee finds that H.R. 5605 would result in no new or increased budget authority, entitlement authority, or tax expenditures or revenues.

### Congressional Budget Office Estimate

Pursuant to clause 3(c)(3) of rule XIII, the following is the cost estimate provided by the Congressional Budget Office pursuant to section 402 of the Congressional Budget Act of 1974:

U.S. Congress, Congressional Budget Office,
Washington, DC, June 6, 2018.
Hon. Greg Walden,

Chairman, Committee on Energy and Commerce, House of Representatives, Washington, DC.

Dear Mr. Chairman: The Congressional Budget Office has prepared the enclosed document with cost estimates for the opioid-related legislation ordered to be reported on May 9 and May 17, 2018.

If you wish further details on this estimate, we will be pleased to provide them. The CBO staff contacts are Tom Bradley and Chad Chirico.

Sincerely,

Mark P. Hadley
(For Keith Hall, Director).

## Opioid Legislation

Summary: On May 9 and May 17, 2018, the House Committee on Energy and Commerce ordered 59 bills to be reported related to the nation's response to the opioid epidemic. Generally, the bills would:

- Provide grants to facilities and providers that treat people with substance use disorders,
- Direct various agencies within the Department of Health and Human Services (HHS) to explore nonopioid approaches to treating pain and to educate providers about those alternatives,
- Modify requirements under Medicaid and Medicare for prescribing controlled substances,
- Expand Medicaid coverage for substance abuse treatment, and
- Direct the Food and Drug Administration (FDA) to modify its oversight of opioid drugs and other medications that are used to manage pain.

Because of the large number of related bills ordered reported by the Committee, CBO is publishing a single comprehensive document that includes estimates for each piece of legislation.

CBO estimates that enacting 20 of the bills would affect direct spending, and 2 of the bills would affect revenues; therefore, pay- as-you-go procedures apply for those bills.

CBO estimates that enacting H.R. 4998, the Health Insurance for Former Foster Youth Act, would increase net direct spending by more than $2.5 billion and on-budget deficits by more than $5 billion in at least one of the four consecutive 10-year periods beginning in 2029. None of the remaining 58 bills included in this estimate would increase net direct spending by more than $2.5 billion or on-budget deficits by more than $5 billion in any of the four consecutive 10-year periods beginning in 2029.

One of the bills reviewed for this document, H.R. 5795, would impose both intergovernmental and private-sector mandates as defined in the Unfunded Mandates Reform Act (UMRA). CBO estimates that the costs of those mandates on public and private entities would fall below the thresholds in UMRA ($80 million and $160 million, respectively, in 2018, adjusted annually for inflation). Five bills, H.R. 5228, H.R. 5333, H.R. 5554, H.R. 5687, and H.R. 5811, would impose private sector mandates as defined in UMRA. CBO estimates that the costs of the mandates in three of the bills (H.R. 5333, H.R. 5554, and H.R. 5811) would not exceed the UMRA threshold for private entities. Because CBO is uncertain how federal agencies would implement new authority granted in the other two bills, H.R. 5228 and H.R. 5687, CBO cannot determine whether the costs of those mandates would exceed the UMRA threshold.

Estimated cost to the Federal Government: The estimates in this document do not include the effects of interactions among the bills. If all 59 bills were combined and enacted as one piece of legislation, the budgetary effects would be different from the sum of the estimates in this document, although CBO expects that any such differences would be small. The costs of this legislation fall within budget functions 550 (health), 570 (Medicare), 750 (administration of justice), and 800 (general government). Basis of estimate: For this estimate, CBO assumes that all of the legislation will be enacted late in 2018 and that authorized and estimated amounts will be appropriated each year. Outlays for discretionary programs are estimated based on historical spending patterns for similar programs.

***Uncertainty***

CBO aims to produce estimates that generally reflect the middle of a range of the most likely budgetary outcomes that would result if the legislation was enacted. Because data on the utilization of mental health and substance abuse treatment under Medicaid and Medicare is scarce, CBO cannot precisely predict how patients or providers would respond to some policy changes or what budgetary effects would result. In addition, several of the bills would give the Department of Health and Human Services (HHS) considerable latitude in designing and implementing policies. Budgetary effects could differ from those provided in CBO's analyses depending on those decisions.

## Direct Spending and Revenues

Table 1 lists the 22 bills of the 59 ordered to be reported that would affect direct spending or revenues.

Legislation Primarily Affecting Medicaid. The following nine bills would affect direct spending for the Medicaid program.

**Table 1. Estimated changes in mandatory spending and revenues**

| | By fiscal year, in millions of dollars— | | | | | | | | | | | | |
|---|---|---|---|---|---|---|---|---|---|---|---|---|---|
| | 2018 | 2019 | 2020 | 2021 | 2022 | 2023 | 2024 | 2025 | 2026 | 2027 | 2028 | 2019–2023 | 2019–2028 |
| | INCREASES OR DECREASES (−) IN DIRECT SPENDING | | | | | | | | | | | | |
| Legislation Primarily Affecting Medicaid: | | | | | | | | | | | | | |
| H.R. 1925, At-Risk Youth Medicaid Protection Act of 2017 | 0 | * | 5 | 5 | 5 | 10 | 10 | 10 | 10 | 10 | 10 | 25 | 75 |
| H.R. 4998, Health Insurance for Former Foster Youth Act | 0 | 0 | 0 | 0 | 0 | * | 10 | 21 | 33 | 46 | 61 | * | 171 |
| H.R. 5477, Rural Development of Opioid Capacity Services Act | 0 | 13 | 35 | 58 | 68 | 83 | 27 | 9 | 3 | 3 | 3 | 256 | 301 |
| H.R. 5583, a bill to amend title XI of the Social Security Act to require States to annually report on certain adult health quality measures, and for other purposes | 0 | * | * | * | * | * | * | * | * | * | * | * | * |
| H.R. 5797, IMD CARE Act | 0 | 38 | 158 | 251 | 265 | 279 | 0 | 0 | 0 | 0 | 0 | 991 | 991 |
| H.R. 5799, Medicaid DRUG Improvement Act [a] | 0 | * | * | 1 | 1 | 1 | 1 | 1 | 1 | 1 | 1 | 2 | 5 |
| H.R. 5801 Medicaid Providers Are Required To Note Experiences in Record Systems to Help In-Need Patients (PARTNERSHIP) Act [a] | 0 | * | * | * | * | * | * | * | * | * | * | * | * |
| H.R. 5808, Medicaid Pharmaceutical Home Act of 2018 [a] | 0 | * | −1 | −1 | −1 | −1 | −2 | −2 | −2 | −2 | −2 | −4 | −13 |
| H.R. 5810, Medicaid Health HOME Act | 0 | 94 | 58 | 62 | 56 | 52 | 48 | 43 | 38 | 32 | 25 | 323 | 509 |
| Legislation Primarily Affecting Medicare: | | | | | | | | | | | | | |
| H.R. 3528, Every Prescription Conveyed Securely Act | 0 | 0 | 0 | −24 | −35 | −33 | −30 | −33 | −32 | −31 | −32 | −92 | −250 |
| H.R. 4841, Standardizing Electronic Prior Authorization for Safe Prescribing Act of 2018 | 0 | 0 | 0 | * | * | * | * | * | * | * | * | * | * |
| H.R. 5603, Access to Telehealth Services for Opioid Use Disorders Act | 0 | 2 | * | * | * | 1 | 1 | 1 | 2 | 2 | 2 | 3 | 11 |
| H.R. 5605, Advancing High Quality Treatment for Opioid Use Disorders in Medicare Act | 0 | 0 | 0 | 15 | 26 | 24 | 23 | 23 | 10 | 1 | * | 65 | 122 |
| H.R. 5675, a bill to amend title XVIII of the Social Security Act to require prescription drug plan sponsors under the Medicare program to establish drug management programs for at-risk beneficiaries | 0 | 0 | 0 | −6 | −7 | −7 | −7 | −8 | −9 | −9 | −11 | −20 | −64 |
| H.R. 5684, Protecting Seniors From Opioid Abuse Act | 0 | 0 | 0 | * | * | * | * | * | * | * | * | * | * |
| H.R. 5796, Responsible Education Achieves Care and Healthy Outcomes for Users' Treatment Act of 2018 | 0 | 10 | 25 | 50 | 10 | 5 | 0 | 0 | 0 | 0 | 0 | 100 | 100 |
| H.R. 5798, Opioid Screening and Chronic Pain Management Alternatives for Seniors Act | 0 | 0 | * | 1 | 1 | 1 | 1 | 1 | 1 | 1 | 1 | 2 | 5 |
| H.R. 5804, Post-Surgical Injections as an Opioid Alternative Act [a] | 0 | 0 | 25 | 30 | 25 | 20 | 10 | 5 | 0 | 0 | 0 | 100 | 115 |
| H.R. 5809, Postoperative Opioid Prevention Act of 2018 | 0 | 0 | 0 | 0 | 10 | 15 | 20 | 25 | 30 | 35 | 45 | 25 | 180 |
| Legislation Primarily Affecting the Food and Drug Administration: | | | | | | | | | | | | | |
| H.R. 5333, Over-the-Counter Monograph Safety, Innovation, and Reform Act of 2018 [a] | 0 | 0 | * | * | * | * | * | * | * | * | * | * | * |
| | INCREASES OR DECREASES (−) IN REVENUES [b] | | | | | | | | | | | | |
| H.R. 5752, Stop Illicit Drug Importation Act of 2018 | 0 | * | * | * | * | * | * | * | * | * | * | * | * |

Annual amounts may not sum to totals because of rounding. * = between ¥$500,000 and $500,000. Budget authority is equivalent to outlays.

[a] This bill also would affect spending subject to appropriation.

[b] One additional bill, H.R. 5228, the Stop Counterfeit Drugs by Regulating and Enhancing Enforcement Now Act, would have a negligible effect on revenues.

*H.R. 1925, the At-Risk Youth Medicaid Protection Act of 2017,* would require states to suspend, rather than terminate, Medicaid eligibility for juvenile enrollees (generally under 21 years of age) who become inmates of public correctional institutions. States also would have to redetermine those enrollees' Medicaid eligibility before their release and restore their coverage upon release if they qualify for the program. States would be required to process Medicaid applications submitted by or on behalf of juveniles in public correctional institutions who were not enrolled in Medicaid before becoming inmates and ensure that Medicaid coverage is provided when they are released if they are found to be eligible. On the basis of an analysis of juvenile incarceration trends and of the per enrollee spending for Medicaid foster care children, who have a similar health profile to incarcerated juveniles, CBO estimates that implementing the bill would cost $75 million over the 2019–2028 period.

*H.R. 4998, the Health Insurance for Former Foster Youth Act,* would require states to provide Medicaid coverage to adults up to age 25 who had aged out of foster care in any state. Under current law, such coverage is mandatory only if the former foster care youth has aged out in the state in which the individual applies for coverage. The policy also would apply to former foster children who had been in foster care upon turning 14 years of age but subsequently left foster care to enter into a legal guardianship with a kinship caregiver. The provisions would take effect respect for foster youth who turn 18 on or after January 1, 2023. On the basis of spending for Medicaid foster care children and data from the Census Bureau regarding annual migration rates between states, CBO estimates that implementing the bill would cost $171 million over the 2019–2028 period.

*H.R. 5477, the Rural Development of Opioid Capacity Services Act,* would direct the Secretary of HHS to conduct a five-year demonstration to increase the number and ability of providers participating in Medicaid to provide treatment for substance use disorders. On the basis of an analysis of federal and state spending for treatment of substance use disorders and the prevalence of such disorders, CBO estimates that enacting the bill would increase direct spending by $301 million over the 2019–2028 period.

*H.R. 5583, a bill to amend title XI of the Social Security Act to require States to annually report on certain adult health quality measures, and for other purposes,* would require states to include behavioral health indicators in their annual reports on the quality of care under Medicaid. Although the bill would add a requirement for states, CBO estimates that its enactment would not have a significant budgetary effect because most states have systems in place for reporting such measures to the federal government.

*H.R. 5797, the IMD CARE Act,* would expand Medicaid coverage for people with opioid use disorder who are in institutions for mental disease (IMDs) for up to 30 days per year. Under a current-law policy known as the IMD exclusion, the federal government generally does not make matching payments to state Medicaid programs for most services provided by IMDs to adults between the ages of 21 and 64. Recent administrative changes have made federal financing for IMDs available in limited circumstances, but the statutory prohibition remains in place. CBO analyzed several data sets, primarily those collected by the Substance Abuse and Mental Health Services Administration (SAMHSA), to estimate current federal spending under Medicaid for IMD services and to estimate spending under H.R. 5797. Using that analysis, CBO estimates that enacting H.R. 5797 would increase direct spending by $991 million over the 2019–2028 period.

*H.R. 5799, the Medicaid DRUG Improvement Act,* would require state Medicaid programs to implement additional reviews of opioid prescriptions, monitor concurrent prescribing of opioids and certain other drugs, and monitor use of antipsychotic drugs by children. CBO estimates that the bill would increase direct spending by $5 million over the 2019–2028 period to cover the administrative costs of complying with those requirements. On the basis of stakeholder feedback, CBO expects that the bill would not have a significant effect on Medicaid spending for prescription drugs because many of the bill's requirements would duplicate current efforts to curb opioid and antipsychotic drug use. (If enacted, H.R. 5799 also would affect spending subject to appropriation; CBO has not completed an estimate of that amount.)

*H.R. 5801, the Medicaid Providers Are Required To Note Experiences in Record Systems to Help-In-Need Patients (PARTNERSHIP) Act,* would require providers who are permitted to prescribe controlled substances and who participate in Medicaid to query prescription drug monitoring programs (PDMPs) before prescribing controlled substances to Medicaid patients. PDMPs are statewide electronic databases that collect data on controlled substances dispensed in the state. The bill also would require PDMPs to comply with certain data and system criteria, and it would provide additional federal matching funds to certain states to help cover administrative costs. On the basis of a literature review and stakeholder feedback, CBO estimates that the net budgetary effect of enacting H.R. 5801 would be insignificant. Costs for states to come into compliance with the systems and administrative requirements would be roughly offset by savings from small reductions in the number of controlled substances paid for by Medicaid under the proposal. (If enacted, H.R. 5801 also would affect spending subject to appropriation; CBO has not completed an estimate of that amount.)

*H.R. 5808, the Medicaid Pharmaceutical Home Act of 2018,* would require state Medicaid programs to operate pharmacy programs that would identify people at high risk of abusing controlled substances and require those patients to use a limited number of providers and pharmacies. Although nearly all state Medicaid programs currently meet such a requirement, a small number of high-risk Medicaid beneficiaries are not now monitored. Based on an analysis of information about similar state and federal programs, CBO estimates that net Medicaid spending under the bill would decrease by $13 million over the 2019–2028 period. That amount represents a small increase in administrative costs and a small reduction in the number of controlled substances paid for by Medicaid under the proposal. (If enacted, H.R. 5808 also would affect spending subject to appropriation; CBO has not completed an estimate of that amount.)

*H.R. 5810, the Medicaid Health HOME Act,* would allow states to receive six months of enhanced federal Medicaid funding for programs that coordinate care for people with substance use disorders. Based on enrollment and spending data from states that currently participate in Medicaid's Health Homes program, CBO estimates that the expansion would cost approximately $469 million over the 2019–2028 period. The bill also would require states to cover all FDA-approved drugs used in medication-assisted treatment for five years, although states could seek a waiver from that requirement. (Medication-assisted treatment combines behavioral therapy and pharmaceutical treatment for substance use disorders.) Under current law, states already cover most FDA-approved drugs used in such programs in some capacity, although a few exclude methadone dispensed by opioid treatment programs. CBO estimates that a small share of those states would begin to cover methadone if this bill was enacted at a federal cost of about $39 million over the 2019–2028 period. In sum, CBO estimates that the enacting H.R. 5810 would increase direct spending by $509 million over the 2019–2028 period.

Legislation Primarily Affecting Medicare. The following ten bills would affect direct spending for the Medicare program.

*H.R. 3528, the Every Prescription Conveyed Securely Act,* would require prescriptions for controlled substances covered under Medicare Part D to be transmitted electronically, starting on January 1, 2021. Based on CBO's analysis of prescription drug spending, spending for controlled substances is a small share of total drug spending. CBO also assumes a small share of those prescriptions would not be filled because they are not converted to an electronic format. Therefore, CBO expects that enacting H.R. 3528 would reduce the number of prescriptions filled and estimates that Medicare spending would be reduced by $250 million over the 2019–2028 period.

*H.R. 4841, the Standardizing Electronic Prior Authorization for Safe Prescribing Act of 2018,* would require health care professionals to submit prior authorization requests electronically, starting on January 1, 2021, for drugs covered under Medicare Part D. Taking into account that many prescribers already use electronic methods to submit such requests, CBO estimates that enacting H.R. 4841 would not significantly affect direct spending for Part D.

*H.R. 5603, the Access to Telehealth Services for Opioid Use Disorders Act,* would permit the Secretary of HHS to lift current geographic and other restrictions on coverage of telehealth services under Medicare for treatment of substance use disorders or co-occurring mental health disorders. Under the bill, the Secretary of HHS would be directed to encourage other payers to coordinate payments for opioid use disorder treatments and to evaluate the extent to which the demonstration reduces hospitalizations, increases the use of medication-assisted treatments, and improves the health outcomes of individuals with opioid use disorders during and after the demonstration. Based on current use of Medicare telehealth services for treatment of substance use disorders, CBO estimates that expanding that coverage would increase direct spending by $11 million over the 2019–2028 period.

*H.R. 5605, the Advancing High Quality Treatment for Opioid Use Disorders in Medicare Act,* would establish a five-year demonstration program to increase access to treatment for opioid use disorder. The demonstration would provide incentive payments and funding for care management services based on criteria such as patient engagement, use of evidence-based treatments, and treatment length and intensity. Under the bill, the Secretary of HHS would be directed to encourage other payers to coordinate payments for opioid use disorder treatments and to evaluate the extent to which the demonstration reduces hospitalizations, increases the use of medication-assisted treatments, and improves the health outcomes of individuals with opioid use disorders during and after the demonstration. Based on historical utilization of opioid use disorder treatments and projected spending on incentive payments and care management fees, CBO estimates that increased use of treatment services and the demonstration's incentive payments would increase direct spending by $122 million over the 2019–2028 period.

*H.R. 5675, a bill to amend title XVIII of the Social Security Act to require prescription drug plan sponsors under the Medicare program to establish drug management programs for at-risk beneficiaries,* would require Part D prescription drug plans to provide drug management programs for Medicare beneficiaries who are at risk for prescription drug abuse. (Under current law, Part D plans are permitted but not required to establish such programs as of 2019.) Based on an analysis of the number of plans currently providing those programs, CBO estimates that enacting H.R. 5675 would lower federal spending by $64 million over the 2019–2028 period by reducing the number of prescriptions filled and Medicare's payments for controlled substances.

*H.R. 5684, the Protecting Seniors From Opioid Abuse Act,* would expand medication therapy management programs under Medicare Part D to include beneficiaries who are at risk for prescription drug abuse. Because relatively few beneficiaries would be affected by this bill, CBO estimates that its enactment would not significantly affect direct spending for Part D.

*H.R. 5796, the Responsible Education Achieves Care and Healthy Outcomes for Users' Treatment Act of 2018,* would allow the Secretary of HHS to award grants to certain organizations that provide technical assistance and education to high-volume prescribers of opioids. The bill would appropriate $100 million for fiscal year 2019. Based on historical spending patterns for similar activities, CBO estimates that implementing H.R. 5796 would cost $100 million over the 2019–2028 period.

*H.R. 5798, the Opioid Screening and Chronic Pain Management Alternatives for Seniors Act,* would add an assessment of current opioid prescriptions and screening for opioid use disorder to the Welcome to Medicare Initial Preventive Physical Examination. Based on historical use of the examinations and pain management alternatives, CBO expects that enacting the bill would increase use of pain management services and estimates that direct spending would increase by $5 million over the 2019–2028 period.

*H.R. 5804, the Post-Surgical Injections as an Opioid Alternative Act,* would freeze the Medicare payment rate for certain analgesic injections provided in ambulatory surgical centers (ASCs). (For injections identified by specific billing codes, Medicare would pay the 2016 rate, which is higher than the current rate, during the 2020– 2024 period.) Based on current utilization in the ASC setting, CBO estimates that enacting the legislation would increase direct spending by about $115 million over the 2019–2028 period. (If enacted, H.R. 5804 also would affect spending subject to appropriation; see Table 3.)

*H.R. 5809, the Postoperative Opioid Prevention Act of 2018,* would create an additional payment under Medicare for nonopioid analgesics. Under current law, certain new drugs and devices may receive an additional payment—separate from the bundled payment for a surgical procedure—in outpatient hospital departments and ambulatory surgical centers. The bill would allow nonopioid analgesics to qualify for a five-year period of additional payments. Based on its assessment of current spending for analgesics and on the probability of new nonopioid analgesics coming to market, CBO estimates that H.R. 5809 would increase direct spending by about $180 million over the 2019–2028 period.

Legislation Primarily Affecting the Food and Drug Administration. One bill related to the FDA would affect direct spending.

*H.R. 5333, the Over-the-Counter Monograph Safety, Innovation, and Reform Act of 2018,* would change the way that the FDA regulates the marketing of over-the-counter (OTC) medicines, and it would authorize that agency to grant 18 months of exclusive market protection for certain qualifying OTC drugs, thus delaying the entry of other versions of the same qualifying OTC product. Medicaid currently provides some coverage for OTC medicines, but only if a medicine is the least costly alternative in its drug class. On the basis of stakeholder feedback, CBO expects that delaying the availability of additional OTC versions of a drug would not significantly affect the average net price paid by Medicaid. As a result, CBO estimates that enacting H.R. 5333 would have a negligible effect on the federal budget. (If enacted, H.R. 5333 also would affect spending subject to appropriation; see Table 3.)

Legislation with Revenue Effects. Two bills would affect revenues. However, CBO estimates that one bill, H.R. 5228, the Stop Counterfeit Drugs by Regulating and Enhancing Enforcement Now Act, would have only a negligible effect.

*H.R. 5752, the Stop Illicit Drug Importation Act of 2018,* would amend the Federal Food, Drug, and Cosmetic Act (FDCA) to strengthen the FDA's seizure powers and enhance its authority to detain, refuse, seize, or destroy illegal products offered for import. The legislation would subject more people to debarment under the FDCA and thus increase the potential for violations, and subsequently, the assessment of civil penalties, which are recorded in the budget as revenues. CBO estimates that those collections would result in an insignificant increase in revenues. Because H.R. 5752 would prohibit the importation of drugs that are in the process of being scheduled, it also could reduce amounts collected in customs duties. CBO anticipates that the result would be a negligible decrease in revenues.

With those results taken together, CBO estimates, enacting H.R. 5752 would generate an insignificant net increase in revenues over the 2019–2028 period.

***Spending Subject to Appropriation***

For this document, CBO has grouped bills with spending that would be subject to appropriation into four general categories:

- Bills that would have no budgetary effect,
- Bills with provisions that would authorize specified amounts to be appropriated (see Table 2),
- Bills with provisions for which CBO has estimated an authorization of appropriations (see Table 3), and
- Bills with provisions that would affect spending subject to appropriation for which CBO has not yet completed an estimate.

No Budgetary Effect. CBO estimates that 6 of the 59 bills would have no effect on direct spending, revenues, or spending subject to appropriation.

*H.R. 3192, the CHIP Mental Health Parity Act,* would require all Children's Health Insurance Program (CHIP) plans to cover mental health and substance abuse treatment. In addition, states would not be allowed to impose financial or utilization limits on mental health treatment that are lower than limits placed on physical health treatment. Based on information from the Centers for Medicare and Medicaid Services, CBO estimates that enacting the bill would have no budgetary effect because all CHIP enrollees are already in plans that meet those requirements.

*H.R. 3331, a bill to amend title XI of the Social Security Act to promote testing of incentive payments for behavioral health providers for adoption and use of certified electronic health record technology,* would give the Center for Medicare and Medicaid Innovation (CMMI) explicit authorization to test a program offering incentive payments to behavioral health providers that adopt and use certified electronic health record technology. Because it is already clear to CMMI that it has that authority,

CBO estimates that enacting the legislation would not affect federal spending.

*H.R. 5202, the Ensuring Patient Access to Substance Use Disorder Treatments Act of 2018,* would clarify permission for pharmacists to deliver controlled substances to providers under certain circumstances. Because this provision would codify current practice, CBO estimates that H.R. 5202 would not affect direct spending or revenues during the 2019–2028 period.

*H.R. 5685, the Medicare Opioid Safety Education Act of 2018,* would require the Secretary of HHS to include information on opioid use, pain management, and nonopioid pain management treatments in future editions of *Medicare & You,* the program's handbook for beneficiaries, starting on January 1, 2019. Because H.R. 5685 would add information to an existing administrative document, CBO estimates that enacting the bill would have no budgetary effect.

*H.R. 5686, the Medicare Clear Health Options in Care for Enrollees Act of 2018,* would require prescription drug plans that provide coverage under Medicare Part D to furnish information to beneficiaries about the risks of opioid use and the availability of alternative treatments for pain. CBO estimates that enacting the bill would not affect direct spending because the required activities would not impose significant administrative costs.

*H.R. 5716, the Commit to Opioid Medical Prescriber Accountability and Safety for Seniors Act,* would require the Secretary of HHS on an annual basis to identify high prescribers of opioids and furnish them with information about proper prescribing methods. Because HHS already has the capacity to meet those requirements, CBO estimates that enacting that provision would not impose additional administrative costs on the agency.

Specified Authorizations. Table 2 lists the ten bills that would authorize specified amounts to be appropriated over the 2019–2023 period. Spending from those authorized amounts would be subject to appropriation.

**Table 2. Estimated spending subject to appropriation for bills with specified authorizations**

| | By fiscal year, in millions of dollars— | | | | | | |
|---|---|---|---|---|---|---|---|
| | 2018 | 2019 | 2020 | 2021 | 2022 | 2023 | 2019–2023 |
| INCREASES IN SPENDING SUBJECT TO APPROPRIATION | | | | | | | |
| H.R. 4684, Ensuring Access to Quality Sober Living Act: | | | | | | | |
| Authorization Level | 0 | 3 | 0 | 0 | 0 | 0 | 3 |
| Estimated Outlays | 0 | 1 | 2 | * | * | * | 3 |
| H.R. 5102, Substance Use Disorder Workforce Loan Repayment Act of 2018: | | | | | | | |
| Authorization Level | 0 | 25 | 25 | 25 | 25 | 25 | 125 |
| Estimated Outlays | 0 | 9 | 19 | 23 | 25 | 25 | 100 |
| H.R. 5176, Preventing Overdoses While in Emergency Rooms Act of 2018: | | | | | | | |
| Authorization Level | 0 | 50 | 0 | 0 | 0 | 0 | 50 |
| Estimated Outlays | 0 | 16 | 26 | 6 | 2 | 1 | 50 |
| H.R. 5197, Alternatives to Opioids (ALTO) in the Emergency Department Act: | | | | | | | |
| Authorization Level | 0 | 10 | 10 | 10 | 0 | 0 | 30 |
| Estimated Outlays | 0 | 3 | 8 | 10 | 7 | 2 | 30 |
| H.R. 5261, Treatment, Education, and Community Help to Combat Addiction Act of 2018: | | | | | | | |
| Authorization Level | 0 | 4 | 4 | 4 | 4 | 4 | 20 |
| Estimated Outlays | 0 | 1 | 3 | 4 | 4 | 4 | 16 |
| H.R. 5327, Comprehensive Opioid Recovery Centers Act of 2018: | | | | | | | |
| Authorization Level | 0 | 10 | 10 | 10 | 10 | 10 | 50 |
| Estimated Outlays | 0 | 3 | 8 | 10 | 10 | 10 | 41 |
| H.R. 5329, Poison Center Network Enhancement Act of 2018: | | | | | | | |
| Authorization Level | 0 | 30 | 30 | 30 | 30 | 30 | 151 |
| Estimated Outlays | 0 | 12 | 25 | 29 | 29 | 29 | 125 |
| H.R. 5353, Eliminating Opioid-Related Infectious Diseases Act of 2018: | | | | | | | |
| Authorization Level | 0 | 40 | 40 | 40 | 40 | 40 | 200 |
| Estimated Outlays | 0 | 15 | 34 | 38 | 39 | 40 | 166 |
| H.R. 5580, Surveillance and Testing of Opioids to Prevent Fentanyl Deaths Act of 2018: | | | | | | | |
| Authorization Level | 30 | 30 | 30 | 30 | 30 | 0 | 120 |
| Estimated Outlays | 0 | 11 | 25 | 29 | 29 | 19 | 113 |
| H.R. 5587, Peer Support Communities of Recovery Act: | | | | | | | |
| Authorization Level | 0 | 15 | 15 | 15 | 15 | 15 | 75 |
| Estimated Outlays | 0 | 5 | 13 | 14 | 15 | 15 | 62 |

Annual amounts may not sum to totals because of rounding. * = between zero and $500,000.

*H.R. 4684, the Ensuring Access to Quality Sober Living Act,* would direct the Secretary of HHS to develop and disseminate best practices for organizations that operate housing designed for people recovering from substance use disorders. The bill would authorize a total of $3 million over the 2019–2021 period for that purpose. Based on historical spending patterns for similar activities, CBO estimates that implementing H.R. 4684 would cost $3 million over the 2019–2023 period.

*H.R. 5102, the Substance Use Disorder Workforce Loan Repayment Act of 2018,* would establish a loan repayment program for mental health professionals who practice in areas with few mental health providers or with high rates of death from overdose and would authorize $25 million per year over the 2019–2028 period for that purpose. Based on historical spending patterns for similar activities, CBO estimates that implementing H.R. 5102 would cost $100 million over the 2019–2023 period; the remaining amounts would be spent in years after 2023.

*H.R. 5176, the Preventing Overdoses While in Emergency Rooms Act of 2018,* would require the Secretary of HHS to develop protocols and a grant program for health care providers to address the needs of people who survive a drug overdose, and it would authorize $50 million in 2019 for that purpose. Based on historical spending patterns for similar activities, CBO estimates that implementing H.R. 5176 would cost $50 million over the 2019–2023 period.

*H.R. 5197, the Alternatives to Opioids (ALTO) in the Emergency Department Act,* would direct the Secretary of HHS to carry out a demonstration program for hospitals and emergency departments to develop alternative protocols for pain management that limit the use of opioids and would authorize $10 million annually in grants for fiscal years 2019 through 2021. Based on historical spending patterns for similar programs, CBO estimates that implementing H.R. 5197 would cost $30 million over the 2019–2023 period.

*H.R. 5261, the Treatment, Education, and Community Help to Combat Addiction Act of 2018,* would direct the Secretary of HHS to designate regional centers of excellence to improve the training of health professionals who treat substance use disorders. The bill would authorize $4 million annually for grants to those programs over the 2019–2023 period. Based on historical spending patterns for similar activities, CBO estimates that implementing H.R. 5261 would cost $16 million over the 2019–2023 period; the remaining amounts would be spent in years after 2023.

*H.R. 5327, the Comprehensive Opioid Recovery Centers Act of 2018,* would direct the Secretary of HHS to award grants to at least 10 providers that offer treatment services for people with opioid use disorder, and it would authorize $10 million per year over the 2019–2023 period for that purpose. Based on historical spending patterns for similar activities, CBO estimates that implementing H.R. 5327 would cost $41 million over the 2019–2023 period; the remaining amounts would be spent in years after 2023.

*H.R. 5329, the Poison Center Network Enhancement Act of 2018,* would reauthorize the poison control center toll-free number, national media campaign, and grant program under the Public Health Service Act. Among other actions, H.R. 5329 would increase the share of poison control center funding that could be provided by federal grants. The bill would authorize a total of about $30 million per year over the 2019–2023 period. Based on historical spending patterns for similar activities, CBO estimates that implementing H.R. 5329 would cost $125 million over the 2019–2023 period; the remaining amounts would be spent in years after 2023.

*H.R. 5353, the Eliminating Opioid Related Infectious Diseases Act of 2018,* would amend the Public Health Service Act by broadening the focus of surveillance and education programs from preventing and treating hepatitis C virus to preventing and treating infections associated with injection drug use. It would authorize $40 million per year over 2019–2023 period for that purpose. Based on historical spending patterns for similar activities, CBO estimates that implementing H.R. 5353 would cost $166 million over the 2019–2023 period; the remaining amounts would be spent in years after 2023.

*H.R. 5580, the Surveillance and Testing of Opioids to Prevent Fentanyl Deaths Act of 2018,* would establish a grant program for public health laboratories that conduct testing for fentanyl and other synthetic opioids. It also would direct the Centers for Disease Control and Prevention to expand its drug surveillance program, with a particular focus on collecting data on fentanyl. The bill would authorize a total of $30 million per year over the 2018–2022 period for those activities. Based on historical spending patterns for similar activities, CBO estimates that implementing H.R. 5580 would cost $113 million over the 2019–2023 period; the remaining amounts would be spent in years after 2023.

*H.R. 5587, Peer Support Communities of Recovery Act,* would direct the Secretary of HHS to award grants to nonprofit organizations that support community-based, peer-delivered support, including technical support for the establishment of recovery community organizations, independent, nonprofit groups led by people in recovery and their families. The bill would authorize $15 million per year for the 2019–2023 period. Based on historical spending patterns for similar activities, CBO estimates that implementing H.R. 5587 would cost $62 million over the 2019–2023 period; the remaining amounts would be spent in years after 2023.

Estimated Authorizations. Table 3 shows CBO's estimates of the appropriations that would be necessary to implement 19 of the bills. Spending would be subject to appropriation of those amounts.

*H.R. 449, the Synthetic Drug Awareness Act of 2018,* would require the Surgeon General to report to the Congress on the health effects of synthetic psychoactive drugs on children between the ages of 12 and 18. Based on spending patterns for similar activities, CBO estimates that implementing H.R. 449 would cost approximately $1 million over the 2019–2023 period.

*H.R. 4005, the Medicaid Reentry Act,* would direct the Secretary of HHS to convene a group of stakeholders to develop and report to the Congress on best practices for addressing issues related to health care faced by those returning from incarceration to their communities. The bill also would require the Secretary to issue a letter to state Medicaid directors about relevant demonstration projects. Based on an analysis of anticipated workload, CBO estimates that implementing H.R. 4005 would cost less than $500,000 over the 2018–2023 period.

*H.R. 4275, the Empowering Pharmacists in the Fight Against Opioid Abuse Act,* would require the Secretary of HHS to develop and disseminate materials for training pharmacists, health care practitioners, and the public about the circumstances under which a pharmacist may decline to fill a prescription. Based on historical spending patterns for similar activities, CBO estimates that costs to the federal government for the development and distribution of those materials would not be significant.

*H.R. 5009, Jessie's Law,* would require HHS, in collaboration with outside experts, to develop best practices for displaying information about opioid use disorder in a patient's medical record. HHS also would be required to develop and disseminate written materials annually to health care providers about what disclosures could be made while still complying with federal laws that govern health care privacy. Based on spending patterns for similar activities, CBO estimates that implementing H.R. 5009 would have an insignificant effect on spending over the 2019–2023 period.

*H.R. 5041, the Safe Disposal of Unused Medication Act,* would require hospice programs to have written policies and procedures for the disposal of controlled substances after a patient's death. Certain licensed employees of hospice programs would be permitted to assist in the disposal of controlled substances that were lawfully dispensed. Using information from the Department of Justice (DOJ), CBO estimates that implementing the bill would cost less than $500,000 over the 2019–2023 period.

*H.R. 5272, the Reinforcing Evidence-Based Standards Under Law in Treating Substance Abuse Act of 2018,* would require the newly established National Mental Health and Substance Use Policy Laboratory to issue guidance to applicants for SAMHSA grants that support evidence-based practices. Using information from HHS about the historical cost of similar activities, CBO estimates that enacting this bill would cost approximately $4 million over the 2019–2023 period.

*H.R. 5333, the Over-the-Counter Monograph Safety, Innovation, and Reform Act of 2018,* would change the FDA's oversight of the commercial marketing of OTC medicines and authorize the collection and spending of fees through 2023 to cover the costs of expediting the FDA's administrative procedures for certain regulatory activities relating to OTC products. Under H.R. 5333, CBO estimates, the FDA would assess about $147 million in fees over the 2019–2023 period that could be collected and made available for obligation only to the extent and in the amounts provided in advance in appropriation acts. Because the FDA could spend those fees, CBO estimates that the estimated budget authority for collections and spending would offset each other exactly in each year, although CBO expects that spending initially would lag behind collections.

## Table 3. Estimated spending subject to appropriation for bills with estimated authorizations

| | By fiscal year, in millions of dollars— | | | | | | |
|---|---|---|---|---|---|---|---|
| | 2018 | 2019 | 2020 | 2021 | 2022 | 2023 | 2019–2023 |
| INCREASES IN SPENDING SUBJECT TO APPROPRIATION | | | | | | | |
| H.R. 449, Synthetic Drug Awareness Act of 2018: | | | | | | | |
| Estimated Authorization Level | 0 | * | * | * | 0 | 0 | 1 |
| Estimated Outlays | 0 | * | * | * | 0 | 0 | 1 |
| H.R. 4005, Medicaid Reentry Act: | | | | | | | |
| Estimated Authorization Level | * | * | 0 | 0 | 0 | 0 | * |
| Estimated Outlays | * | * | 0 | 0 | 0 | 0 | * |
| H.R. 4275, Empowering Pharmacists in the Fight Against Opioid Abuse Act: | | | | | | | |
| Estimated Authorization Level | 0 | * | * | * | * | * | * |
| Estimated Outlays | 0 | * | * | * | * | * | * |
| H.R. 5009, Jessie's Law: | | | | | | | |
| Estimated Authorization Level | 0 | * | * | * | * | * | * |
| Estimated Outlays | 0 | * | * | * | * | * | * |
| H.R. 5041, Safe Disposal of Unused Medication Act: | | | | | | | |
| Estimated Authorization Level | 0 | * | * | * | * | * | * |
| Estimated Outlays | 0 | * | * | * | * | * | * |
| H.R. 5272, Reinforcing Evidence-Based Standards Under Law in Treating Substance Abuse Act of 2018: | | | | | | | |
| Estimated Authorization Level | 0 | 1 | 1 | 1 | 1 | 1 | 4 |
| Estimated Outlays | 0 | 1 | 1 | 1 | 1 | 1 | 4 |
| H.R. 5333, Over-the-Counter Monograph Safety, Innovation, and Reform Act of 2018: [a] | | | | | | | |
| Food and Drug Administration: | | | | | | | |
| Collections from fees: | | | | | | | |
| Estimated Authorization Level | 0 | −22 | −22 | −26 | −35 | −42 | −147 |
| Estimated Outlays | 0 | −22 | −22 | −26 | −35 | −42 | −147 |
| Spending of fees: | | | | | | | |
| Estimated Authorization Level | 0 | 22 | 22 | 26 | 35 | 42 | 147 |
| Estimated Outlays | 0 | 6 | 17 | 30 | 44 | 41 | 137 |
| Net effect on FDA: | | | | | | | |
| Estimated Authorization Level | 0 | 0 | 0 | 0 | 0 | 0 | 0 |
| Estimated Outlays | 0 | −17 | −6 | 4 | 9 | * | −10 |
| Government Accountability Office: | | | | | | | |
| Estimated Authorization Level | 0 | 0 | 0 | 0 | 0 | * | * |
| Estimated Outlays | 0 | 0 | 0 | 0 | 0 | * | * |
| **Total, H.R. 5333:** | | | | | | | |
| Estimated Authorization Level | 0 | 0 | 0 | 0 | 0 | * | * |
| Estimated Outlays | 0 | −17 | −6 | 4 | 9 | * | −10 |
| H.R. 5473, Better Pain Management Through Better Data Act of 2018: | | | | | | | |
| Estimated Authorization Level | 0 | * | * | * | * | 0 | 1 |
| Estimated Outlays | 0 | * | * | * | * | * | 1 |
| H.R. 5483, Special Registration for Telemedicine Clarification Act of 2018: | | | | | | | |
| Estimated Authorization Level | 0 | * | * | * | * | * | * |
| Estimated Outlays | 0 | * | * | * | * | * | * |
| H.R. 5554, Animal Drug and Animal Generic Drug User Fee Amendments of 2018: | | | | | | | |
| Collections from fees: | | | | | | | |
| Animal drug fees | 0 | −30 | −31 | −32 | −33 | −34 | −159 |
| Generic animal drug fees | 0 | −18 | −19 | −19 | −20 | −21 | −97 |
| Total, Estimated Authorization Level | 0 | −49 | −50 | −51 | −53 | −55 | −257 |
| Total, Estimated Outlays | 0 | −49 | −50 | −51 | −53 | −55 | −257 |
| Spending of fees: | | | | | | | |
| Animal drug fees | 0 | 30 | 31 | 32 | 33 | 34 | 159 |
| Generic animal drug fees | 0 | 18 | 19 | 19 | 20 | 21 | 97 |
| Total, Estimated Authorization Level | 0 | 49 | 50 | 51 | 53 | 55 | 257 |
| Total, Estimated Outlays | 0 | 39 | 47 | 51 | 52 | 54 | 243 |

| | By fiscal year, in millions of dollars— | | | | | | |
|---|---|---|---|---|---|---|---|
| | 2018 | 2019 | 2020 | 2021 | 2022 | 2023 | 2019–2023 |
| Net changes in fees: | | | | | | | |
| Estimated Authorization Level | 0 | 0 | 0 | 0 | 0 | 0 | 0 |
| Estimated Outlays | 0 | −10 | −3 | * | * | * | −14 |
| Other effects: | | | | | | | |
| Estimated Authorization Level | 0 | 3 | 1 | 1 | 1 | 1 | 6 |
| Estimated Outlays | 0 | 2 | 1 | 1 | 1 | 1 | 6 |
| **Total, H.R. 5554:** | | | | | | | |
| Estimated Authorization Level | 0 | 3 | 1 | 1 | 1 | 1 | 6 |
| Estimated Outlays | 0 | −8 | −2 | 1 | * | * | −8 |
| H.R. 5582, Abuse Deterrent Access Act of 2018: | | | | | | | |
| Estimated Authorization Level | 0 | 0 | * | 0 | 0 | 0 | * |
| Estimated Outlays | 0 | 0 | * | 0 | 0 | 0 | * |
| H.R. 5590, Opioid Addiction Action Plan Act: | | | | | | | |
| Estimated Authorization Level | * | * | * | * | * | * | 2 |
| Estimated Outlays | * | * | * | * | * | * | 2 |
| H.R. 5687, Securing Opioids and Unused Narcotics with Deliberate Disposal and Packaging Act of 2018: | | | | | | | |
| Estimated Authorization Level | 0 | * | * | * | * | * | * |
| Estimated Outlays | 0 | * | * | * | * | * | * |
| H.R. 5715, Strengthening Partnerships to Prevent Opioid Abuse Act: | | | | | | | |
| Estimated Authorization Level | 0 | 2 | 2 | 2 | 2 | 2 | 9 |
| Estimated Outlays | 0 | 2 | 2 | 2 | 2 | 2 | 9 |
| H.R. 5789, a bill to require the Secretary of Health and Human Services to issue guidance to improve care for infants with neonatal abstinence syndrome and their mothers, and to require the Comptroller General of the United States to conduct a study on gaps in Medicaid coverage for pregnant and postpartum women with substance use disorder: | | | | | | | |
| Estimated Authorization Level | 0 | 2 | 0 | 0 | 0 | 0 | 2 |
| Estimated Outlays | 0 | 2 | 0 | 0 | 0 | 0 | 2 |
| H.R. 5795, Overdose Prevention and Patient Safety Act: | | | | | | | |
| Estimated Authorization Level | 0 | 1 | 0 | 0 | 0 | 0 | 1 |
| Estimated Outlays | 0 | 1 | 0 | 0 | 0 | 0 | 1 |
| H.R. 5800, Medicaid IMD ADDITIONAL INFO Act: | | | | | | | |
| Estimated Authorization Level | 0 | 1 | 0 | 0 | 0 | 0 | 1 |
| Estimated Outlays | 0 | * | * | 0 | 0 | 0 | 1 |
| H.R. 5804, Post-Surgical Injections as an Opioid Alternative Act: [a] | | | | | | | |
| Estimated Authorization Level | 0 | 0 | 0 | 0 | 1 | 1 | 1 |
| Estimated Outlays | 0 | 0 | 0 | 0 | 1 | 1 | 1 |
| H.R. 5811, a bill to amend the Federal Food, Drug, and Cosmetic Act with respect to postapproval study requirements for certain controlled substances, and for other purposes: | | | | | | | |
| Estimated Authorization Level | 0 | * | * | * | * | * | * |
| Estimated Outlays | 0 | * | * | * | * | * | * |

Annual amounts may not sum to totals because of rounding. * = between ¥$500,000 and $500,000.

[a] This bill also would affect mandatory spending (see Table 1).

Assuming appropriation action consistent with the bill, CBO estimates that implementing H.R. 5333 would reduce net discretionary outlays by $10 million over the 2019–2023 period, primarily because of that lag. The bill also would require the Government Accountability Office to study exclusive market protections for certain qualifying OTC drugs authorized by the bill—a provision that CBO estimates would cost less than $500,000. (If enacted, H.R. 5333 also would affect mandatory spending; see Table 1.)

*H.R. 5473, the Better Pain Management Through Better Data Act of 2018,* would require that the FDA conduct a public meeting and issue guidance to industry addressing data collection and labeling for medical products that reduce pain while enabling the reduction, replacement, or avoidance of oral opioids. Using information from the agency, CBO estimates that implementing H.R. 5473 would cost about $1 million over the 2019–2023 period.

*H.R. 5483, the Special Registration for Telemedicine Clarification Act of 2018,* would direct DOJ, within one year of the bill's enactment, to issue regulations concerning the practice of telemedicine (for remote diagnosis and treatment of patients). Using information from DOJ, CBO estimates that implementing the bill would cost less than $500,000 over the 2019–2023 period.

*H.R. 5554, the Animal Drug and Animal Generic Drug User Fee Amendments of 2018,* would authorize the FDA to collect and spend fees to cover the cost of expedited approval for the development and marketing of certain drugs for use in animals. The legislation would extend through fiscal year 2023, and make several changes to, the FDA's existing approval processes and fee programs for brand-name and generic veterinary drugs, which expire at the end of fiscal year 2018. CBO estimates that implementing H.R. 5554 would reduce net discretionary outlays by $8 million over the 2019–2023 period, primarily because the spending of fees lags somewhat behind their collection.

Fees authorized under the bill would supplement funds appropriated to cover the FDA's cost of reviewing certain applications and investigational submissions for brand-name and generic drugs for use in animals. Those fees could be collected and made available for obligation only to the extent and in the amounts provided in advance in appropriation acts. Under H.R. 5554, CBO estimates, the FDA would assess about $257 million in fees over the 2019– 2023 period. Because the FDA could spend those funds, CBO estimates that budget authority for collections and spending would offset each other exactly in each year. CBO estimates that the delay between collecting and spending fees under the reauthorized programs would reduce net discretionary outlays by $14 million over the 2019–2023 period, assuming appropriation actions consistent with the bill.

Enacting H.R. 5554 would increase the FDA's workload because the legislation would expand eligibility for conditional approval for certain drugs. The agency's administrative costs also would increase because of regulatory activities required by a provision concerning petitions for additives intended for use in animal food. H.R. 5554 also would require the FDA to publish guidance or produce regulations on a range of topics, transmit a report to the Congress, and hold public meetings. CBO expects that the costs associated with those activities would not be covered by fees, and it estimates that implementing such provisions would cost $6 million over the 2019–2023 period.

*H.R. 5582, the Abuse Deterrent Access Act of 2018,* would require the Secretary of HHS to report to the Congress on existing barriers to access to "abuse-deterrent opioid formulations" by Medicare Part C and D beneficiaries. Such formulations make the drugs more difficult to dissolve for injection, for example, and thus can impede their abuse. Assuming the availability of appropriated funds and based on historical spending patterns for similar activities, CBO estimates that implementing the legislation would cost less than $500,000 over the 2019–2023 period.

*H.R. 5590, the Opioid Addiction Action Plan Act,* would require the Secretary of HHS to develop an action plan by January 1, 2019, for increasing access to medication-assisted treatment among Medicare and Medicaid enrollees. The bill also would require HHS to convene a stakeholder meeting and issue a request for information within three months of enactment, and to submit a report to the Congress by June 1, 2019. Based on historical spending patterns for similar activities, CBO estimates that implementing H.R. 5590 would cost approximately $2 million over the 2019–2023 period.

*H.R. 5687, the Securing Opioids and Unused Narcotics with Deliberate Disposal and Packaging Act of 2018,* would permit the FDA to require certain packaging and disposal technologies, controls, or measures to mitigate the risk of abuse and misuse of drugs. Based on information from the FDA, CBO estimates that implementing H.R. 5687 would not significantly affect spending over the 2019–2023 period. This bill would also require that the GAO study the effectiveness and use of packaging technologies for controlled substances—a provision that CBO estimates would cost less than $500,000.

*H.R. 5715, the Strengthening Partnerships to Prevent Opioid Abuse Act,* would require the Secretary of HHS to establish a secure Internet portal to allow HHS, Medicare Advantage plans, and Medicare Part D plans to exchange information about fraud, waste, and abuse among providers and suppliers no later than two years after enactment. H.R. 5715 also would require organizations with Medicare Advantage contracts to submit information on investigations related to providers suspected of prescribing large volumes of opioids through a process established by the Secretary no later than January 2021. Based on historical spending patterns for similar activities, CBO estimates that implementing H.R. 5715 would cost approximately $9 million over the 2019–2023 period.

*H.R. 5789, a bill to require the Secretary of Health and Human Services to issue guidance to improve care for infants with neonatal abstinence syndrome and their mothers, and to require the Comptroller General of the United States to conduct a study on gaps in Medicaid coverage for pregnant and postpartum women with substance use disorder,* would direct the Secretary of HHS to issue guidance to states on best practices under Medicaid and CHIP for treating infants with neonatal abstinence syndrome. H.R. 5789 also would direct the Government Accountability Office to study Medicaid coverage for pregnant and postpartum women with substance use disorders. Based on information from HHS and historical spending patterns for similar activities, CBO estimates that enacting H.R. 5789 would cost approximately $2 million over the 2019– 2023 period.

*H.R. 5795, the Overdose Prevention and Patient Safety Act,* would amend the Public Health Service Act so that requirements pertaining to the confidentiality and disclosure of medical records relating to substance use disorders align with the provisions of the Health Insurance Portability and Accountability Act of 1996. The bill would require the Office of the Secretary of HHS to issue regulations prohibiting discrimination based on data disclosed from such medical records, to issue regulations requiring covered entities to provide written notice of privacy practices, and to develop model training programs and materials for health care providers and patients and their families. Based on spending patterns for similar activities, CBO estimates that implementing H.R. 5795 would cost approximately $1 million over the 2019–2023 period.

*H.R. 5800, Medicaid IMD ADDITIONAL INFO Act,* would direct the Medicaid and CHIP Payment and Access Commission to study institutions for mental diseases in a representative sample of states. Based on information from the commission about the cost of similar work, CBO estimates that implementing H.R. 5800 would cost about $1 million over the 2019–2023 period.

*H.R. 5804, the Post-Surgical Injections as an Opioid Alternative Act,* would freeze the Medicare payment rate for certain analgesic injections provided in ambulatory surgical centers. The bill also would mandate two studies of Medicare coding and payments arising from enactment of this legislation. Based on the cost of similar activities, CBO estimates that those reports would cost $1 million over the 2019–2023 period. (If enacted, H.R. 5804 also would affect mandatory spending; see Table 1.)

*H.R. 5811, a bill to amend the Federal Food, Drug, and Cosmetic Act with respect to postapproval study requirements for certain controlled substances, and for other purposes,* would allow the FDA to require that pharmaceutical manufacturers study certain drugs after they are approved to assess any potential reduction in those drugs' effectiveness for the conditions of use prescribed, recommended, or suggested in labeling. CBO anticipates that implementing H.R. 5811 would not significantly affect the FDA's costs over the 2019–2023 period.

Other Authorizations. The following nine bills would increase authorization levels, but CBO has not completed estimates of amounts. All authorizations would be subject to future appropriation action.

- H.R. 4284, Indexing Narcotics, Fentanyl, and Opioids Act of 2017
- H.R. 5002, Advancing Cutting Edge Research Act
- H.R. 5228, Stop Counterfeit Drugs by Regulating and Enhancing Enforcement Now Act (see Table 1 for an estimate of the revenue effects of H.R. 5228)
- H.R. 5752, Stop Illicit Drug Importation Act of 2018 (see Table 1 for an estimate of the revenue effects of H.R. 5752)
- H.R. 5799, Medicaid DRUG Improvement Act (see Table 1 for an estimate of the direct spending effects of H.R. 5799)
- H.R. 5801, Medicaid Providers and Pharmacists Are Required to Note Experiences in Record Systems to Help In-Need Patients (PARTNERSHIP) Act (see Table 1 for an estimate of the direct spending effects of H.R. 5801)
- H.R. 5806, 21st Century Tools for Pain and Addiction Treatments Act
- H.R. 5808, Medicaid Pharmaceutical Home Act of 2018 (see Table 1 for an estimate of the direct spending effects of H.R. 5808)
- H.R. 5812, Creating Opportunities that Necessitate New and Enhanced Connections That Improve Opioid Navigation Strategies Act (CONNECTIONS)

Act Pay-As-You-Go considerations: The Statutory Pay-As-You-Go Act of 2010 establishes budget-reporting and enforcement procedures for legislation affecting direct spending or revenues. Twenty-two of the bills discussed in this document contain direct spending or revenues and are subject to pay-as-you-go procedures. Details about the amount of direct spending and revenues in those bills can be found in Table 1.

Increase in long-term direct spending and deficits: CBO estimates that enacting H.R. 4998, the Health Insurance for Former Foster Youth Act, would increase net direct spending by more than $2.5 billion and on-budget deficits by more than $5 billion in at least one of the four consecutive 10-year periods beginning in 2029. CBO estimates that none of the remaining 58 bills included in this estimate would increase net direct spending by more than $2.5 billion or on-budget deficits by more than $5 billion in any of the four consecutive 10-year periods beginning in 2029.

Mandates: One of the 59 bills included in this document, H.R. 5795, would impose both intergovernmental and private-sector mandates as defined in UMRA. CBO estimates that the costs of that bill's mandates on public and private entities would fall below UMRA's thresholds ($80 million and $160 million, respectively, for public- and private-sector entities in 2018, adjusted annually for inflation).

In addition, five bills would impose private-sector mandates as defined in UMRA. CBO estimates that the costs of the mandates in three of those bills (H.R. 5333, H.R. 5554, and H.R. 5811) would fall below the UMRA threshold. Because CBO does not know how federal agencies would implement new authority granted in the other two of those five bills, H.R. 5228 and 5687, CBO cannot determine whether the costs of their mandates would exceed the threshold.

For large entitlement grant programs, including Medicaid and CHIP, UMRA defines an increase in the stringency of conditions on states or localities as an intergovernmental mandate if the affected governments lack authority to offset those costs while continuing to provide required services. Because states possess significant flexibility to alter their responsibilities within Medicaid and CHIP, the requirements imposed by various bills in the markup on state administration of those programs would not constitute mandates as defined in UMRA.

### *Mandates Affecting Public and Private Entities*

*H.R. 5795, the Overdose Prevention and Patient Safety Act,* would impose intergovernmental and private-sector mandates by requiring entities that provide treatment for substance use disorders to notify patients of their privacy rights and also to notify patients in the event that the confidentiality of their records is breached. In certain circumstances, H.R. 5795 also would prohibit public and private entities from denying entry to treatment on the basis of information in patient health records. Those requirements would either supplant or narrowly expand responsibilities under existing law, and compliance with them would not impose significant additional costs. CBO estimates that the costs of the mandates would fall below the annual thresholds established in UMRA.

### *Mandates Affecting Private Entities*

Five bills included in this document would impose private-sector mandates:

*H.R. 5228, the Stop Counterfeit Drugs by Regulating and Enhancing Enforcement Now Act,* would require drug distributors to cease distributing any drug that the Secretary of HHS determines might present an imminent or substantial hazard to public health. CBO cannot determine what drugs could be subject to such an order nor can it determine how private entities would respond. Consequently, CBO cannot determine whether the aggregate cost of the mandate would exceed the annual threshold for private-sector mandates.

*H.R. 5333, the Over-the-Counter Monograph Safety, Innovation, and Reform Act of 2018,* would require developers and manufacturers of OTC drugs to pay certain fees to the FDA. CBO estimates that about $30 million would be collected each year, on average, for a total of $147 million over the 2019–2023 period. Those amounts would not exceed the annual threshold for private-sector mandates in any year during that period.

*H.R. 5554, the Animal Drug and Animal Generic Drug User Fee Amendments of 2018,* would require developers and manufacturers of brand-name and generic veterinary drugs to pay application, product, establishment, and sponsor fees to the FDA. CBO estimates that about $51 million would be collected annually, on average, for a total of $257 million over the 2019–2023 period. Those amounts would not exceed the annual threshold for private-sector mandates in any year during that period.

*H.R. 5687, the Securing Opioids and Unused Narcotics with Deliberate Disposal and Packaging Act of 2018,* would permit the

Secretary of HHS to require drug developers and manufacturers to implement new packaging and disposal technology for certain drugs. Based on information from the agency, CBO expects that the Secretary would use the new regulatory authority provided in the bill; however, it is uncertain how or when those requirements would be implemented. Consequently, CBO cannot determine whether the aggregate cost of the mandate would exceed the annual threshold for private entities.

*H.R. 5811, a bill to amend the Federal Food, Drug, and Cosmetic Act with respect to postapproval study requirements for certain controlled substances, and for other purposes,* would expand an existing mandate that requires drug developers to conduct postapproval studies or clinical trials for certain drugs. Under current law, in certain instances, the FDA can require studies or clinical trials after a drug has been approved. H.R. 5811 would permit the FDA to use that authority if the reduction in a drug's effectiveness meant that its benefits no longer outweighed its costs. CBO estimates that the incremental cost of the mandate would fall below the annual threshold established in UMRA because of the small number of drugs affected and the narrow expansion of the authority that exists under current law.

None of the remaining 53 bills included in this document would impose an intergovernmental or private-sector mandate.

Previous CBO estimate: On June 6, 2018, CBO issued an estimate for seven opioid-related bills ordered reported by the House Committee on Ways and Means on May 16, 2018. Two of those bills contain provisions that are identical or similar to the legislation ordered reported by the Committee on Energy and Commerce, and for those provisions, CBO's estimates are the same.

In particular, five bills listed in this estimate contain provisions that are identical or similar to those in several sections of H.R. 5773, the Preventing Addiction for Susceptible Seniors Act of 2018:

- H.R. 5675, which would require prescription drug plans to implement drug management programs, is identical to section 2 of H.R. 5773.

- H.R. 4841, regarding electronic prior authorization for prescriptions under Medicare's Part D, is similar to section 3 of H.R. 5773.
- H.R. 5715, which would mandate the creation of a new Internet portal to allow various stakeholders to exchange information, is identical to section 4 of H.R. 5773.
- H.R. 5684, which would expand medication therapy management, is the same as section 5 of H.R. 5773.
- H.R. 5716, regarding prescriber notification, is identical to section 6 of H.R. 5773.

In addition, in this estimate, a provision related to Medicare beneficiary education in H.R. 5686, the Medicare Clear Health Options in Care for Enrollees Act of 2018, is the same as a provision in section 2 of H.R. 5775, the Providing Reliable Options for Patients and Educational Resources Act of 2018, in CBO's estimate for the Committee on Ways and Means.

Estimate prepared by: Federal Costs: Rebecca Yip (Centers for Disease Control and Prevention), Mark Grabowicz (Drug Enforcement Agency), Julia Christensen, Ellen Werble (Food and Drug Administration), Emily King, Andrea Noda, Lisa Ramirez-Branum, Robert Stewart (Medicaid and Children's Health Insurance Program), Philippa Haven, Lara Robillard, Colin Yee, Rebecca Yip (Medicare), Philippa Haven (National Institutes of Health), Alice Burns, Andrea Noda (Office of the Secretary of the Department of Health and Human Services), Philippa Haven, Lori Housman, Emily King (Substance Abuse and Mental Health Services Administration, Health Resources and Services Administration); Federal Revenues: Jacob Fabian, Peter Huether, and Cecilia Pastrone; Fact Checking: Zachary Byrum and Kate Kelly; Mandates: Andrew Laughlin.

Estimate reviewed by: Tom Bradley, Chief, Health Systems and Medicare Cost Estimates Unit; Chad M. Chirico, Chief, Low-Income Health Programs and Prescription Drugs Cost Estimates Unit; Sarah Masi, Special Assistant for Health; Susan Willie, Chief, Mandates Unit; Leo Lex,

Deputy Assistant Director for Budget Analysis; Theresa A. Gullo, Assistant Director for Budget Analysis.

## FEDERAL MANDATES STATEMENT

The Committee adopts as its own the estimate of Federal mandates prepared by the Director of the Congressional Budget Office pursuant to section 423 of the Unfunded Mandates Reform Act.

## STATEMENT OF GENERAL PERFORMANCE GOALS AND OBJECTIVES

Pursuant to clause 3(c)(4) of rule XIII, the general performance goal or objective of this legislation is to work with eligible entities, including Quality Improvement Organizations, to instruct the Centers for Medicare and Medicaid Services (CMS) to create a demonstration project to test new ways to treat opioid use disorder among the Medicare population. This model includes the development of measures to evaluate the quality and outcomes of treatment.

## DUPLICATION OF FEDERAL PROGRAMS

Pursuant to clause 3(c)(5) of rule XIII, no provision H.R. 5605 is known to be duplicative of another Federal program, including any program that was included in a report to Congress pursuant to section 21 of Public Law 111–139 or the most recent Catalog of Federal Domestic Assistance.

## Committee Cost Estimate

Pursuant to clause 3(d)(1) of rule XIII, the Committee adopts as its own the cost estimate prepared by the Director of the Congressional Budget Office pursuant to section 402 of the Congressional Budget Act of 1974.

## Earmark, Limited Tax Benefits, and Limited Tariff Benefits

Pursuant to clause 9(e), 9(f), and 9(g) of rule XXI, the Committee finds that H.R. 5605 contains no earmarks, limited tax benefits, or limited tariff benefits.

## Disclosure of Directed Rule Makings

Pursuant to section 3(i) of H. Res. 5, the Committee finds that H.R. 5605 contains no directed rule makings.

## Advisory Committee Statement

No advisory committees within the meaning of section 5(b) of the Federal Advisory Committee Act were created by this legislation.

## Applicability to Legislative Branch

The Committee finds that the legislation does not relate to the terms and conditions of employment or access to public services or accommodations within the meaning of section 102(b)(3) of the Congressional Accountability Act.

## SECTION-BY-SECTION ANALYSIS OF THE LEGISLATION

### Section 1. Short Title

Section 1 provides that the Act may be cited as the Advancing High Quality Treatment for Opioid Use Disorders in Medicare Act.

### Section 2. Opioid Use Treatment Demonstration Program

The Secretary shall implement a five-year demonstration program to increase access to opioid use disorder treatment services and to improve physical and mental health outcomes for beneficiaries.

## CHANGES IN EXISTING LAW MADE BY THE BILL, AS REPORTED

In compliance with clause 3(e) of rule XIII of the Rules of the House of Representatives, changes in existing law made by the bill, as reported, are shown as follows (new matter is printed in italic and existing law in which no change is proposed is shown in roman): Social Security Act Title XVIII—Health Insurance For The Aged And Disabled. Part E—Miscellaneous Provisions

# SEC. 1866F. OPIOID USE DISORDER TREATMENT DEMONSTRATION PROGRAM

(a)IMPLEMENTATION OF 5-YEAR DEMONSTRATION PROGRAM.—

(1) IN GENERAL.—Not later than January 1, 2021, the Secretary shall implement a 5-year demonstration program under this title (in this section referred to as the "Program") to increase access of applicable beneficiaries to opioid use disorder treatment services, improve physical and mental health outcomes for such beneficiaries, and to the extent possible, reduce expenditures under this title. Under the Program, the Secretary shall make payments under subsection (e) to participants (as defined in subsection (c)(1)(A)) for furnishing opioid use disorder treatment services delivered through opioid use disorder care teams, or arranging for such service to be furnished, to applicable beneficiaries participating in the Program.

(2) OPIOID USE DISORDER TREATMENT SERVICES.—For purposes of this section, the term "opioid use disorder treatment services"—

(A) means, with respect to an applicable beneficiary, services that are furnished for the treatment of opioid use disorders and that utilize drugs approved under section 505 of the Federal Food, Drug, and Cosmetic Act for the treatment of opioid use disorders in an outpatient setting; and

(B)includes—

(i) medication assisted treatment;

(ii) treatment planning;

(iii) psychiatric, psychological, or counseling services (or any combination of such services), as appropriate;

(iv) social support services, as appropriate; and

(v) care management and care coordination services, including coordination with other providers of services and suppliers not on an opioid use disorder care team.

(b)PROGRAM DESIGN.—

(1) IN GENERAL.—The Secretary shall design the Program in such a manner to allow for the evaluation of the extent to which the Program accomplishes the following purposes:

(A) Reduces hospitalizations and emergency department visits.

(B) Increases use of medication-assisted treatment for opioid use disorders.

(C) Improves health outcomes of individuals with opioid use disorders, including by reducing the incidence of infectious diseases (such as hepatitis C and HIV).

(D) Does not increase the total spending on items and services under this title.

(E) Reduces deaths from opioid overdose.

(F) Reduces the utilization of inpatient residential treatment.

(2) CONSULTATION.—In designing the Program, including the criteria under subsection (e)(2)(A), the Secretary shall, not later than 3 months after the date of the enactment of this section, consult with specialists in the field of addiction, clinicians in the primary care community, and beneficiary groups.

(c) PARTICIPANTS; OPIOID USE DISORDER CARE TEAMS.—

(1) PARTICIPANTS.—

(A) DEFINITION.—In this section, the term "participant" means an entity or individual—

(i) that is otherwise enrolled under this title and that is—

(I) a physician (as defined in section 1861(r)(1);

(II) a group practice comprised of physicians described in subclause (I);

(III) a hospital outpatient department;

(IV) a federally qualified health center (as defined in section 1861(aa)(4));

(V) a rural health clinic (as defined in section 1861(aa)(2));

(VI) a community mental health center (as defined in section 1861(ff)(3)(B));

(VII) a clinic certified as a certified community behavioral health clinic pursuant to section 223 of the Protecting Access to Medicare Act of 2014; or

(VIII) any other individual or entity specified by the Secretary;

(ii) that applied for and was selected to participate in the Program pursuant to an application and selection process established by the Secretary; and

(iii) that establishes an opioid use disorder care team (as defined in paragraph (2)) through employing or contracting with health care practitioners described in paragraph (2)(A), and uses such team to furnish or arrange for opioid use disorder treatment services in the outpatient setting under the Program

(B) PREFERENCE.—In selecting participants for the Program, the Secretary shall give preference to individuals and entities that are located in areas with a prevalence of opioid use disorders that is higher than the national average prevalence.

(2) OPIOID USE DISORDER CARE TEAMS.—

(A) IN GENERAL.—For purposes of this section, the term "opioid use disorder care team" means a team of health care practitioners established by a participant described in paragraph (1)(A) that—

(i) shall include—

(I) at least one physician (as defined in section 1861(r)(1)) furnishing primary care services or addiction treatment services to an applicable beneficiary; and

(II) at least one eligible practitioner (as defined in paragraph (3)(A)), who may be a physician who meets the criterion in subclause (I); and

(ii) may include other practitioners licensed under State law to furnish psychiatric, psychological, counseling, and social services to applicable beneficiaries.

(B)REQUIREMENTS FOR RECEIPT OF PAYMENT UNDER PROGRAM.—In order to receive payments under subsection (e), each participant in the Program shall—

(i)furnish opioid use disorder treatment services through opioid use disorder care teams to applicable beneficiaries who agree to receive the services;

(ii) meet minimum criteria, as established by the Secretary, for participation through the submission of data and information described in clause (iii); and

(iii) submit to the Secretary, with respect to each applicable beneficiary for whom opioid use disorder treatment services are furnished by the opioid use disorder care team, data with respect to the criteria established under subsection (e)(2)(A) and such other information as the Secretary determines appropriate to monitor and evaluate the Program, to determine if minimum criteria are met under clause (ii), and to determine the incentive payment under subsection (e), in such form, manner, and frequency as specified by the Secretary.

(3) ELIGIBLE PRACTITIONERS; OTHER PROVIDER-RELATED DEFINITIONS AND APPLICATION PROVISIONS.—

(A) ELIGIBLE PRACTITIONERS.—For purposes of this section, the term "eligible practitioner" means a physician or other health care practitioner, such as a nurse practitioner or advanced practice nurse, that—

(i) is enrolled under section 1861(j);

(ii) is authorized to prescribe or dispense narcotic drugs to individuals for maintenance treatment or detoxification treatment; and

(iii) has in effect a registration or waiver in accordance with section 303(g) of the Controlled Substances Act for such purpose and is otherwise in compliance with regulations promulgated by the Substance Abuse and Mental Health Services Administration to carry out such section.

(B) ADDICTION SPECIALISTS.—For purposes of subsection (e)(1)(B)(iv), the term "addiction specialist" means a physician that possesses expert knowledge and skills in addiction medicine, as evidenced by appropriate certification from a specialty body, a certificate of advanced qualification in addiction medicine, or completion of an accredited residency or fellowship in addiction medicine or addiction psychiatry, as determined by the Secretary.

(d)PARTICIPATION OF APPLICABLE BENEFICIARIES.—

(1) APPLICABLE BENEFICIARY DEFINED.—In this section, the term "applicable beneficiary" means an individual who—

(A) is entitled to, or enrolled for, benefits under part A and enrolled for benefits under part B;

(B) is not enrolled in a Medicare Advantage plan under part C;

(C) has a current diagnosis for an opioid use disorder; and

(D) meets such other criteria as the Secretary determines appropriate.

Such term shall include an individual who is dually eligible for benefits under this title and title XIX if such individual satisfies the criteria described in subparagraphs (A) through (D).

(2) VOLUNTARY PARTICIPATION; LIMITATION ON NUMBER OF PARTICIPANTS.—An applicable beneficiary may participate in the Program on a voluntary basis and may terminate participation in the Program at any time. Not more than 20,000 applicable beneficiaries may participate in the Program.

(3) SERVICES.—In order to participate in the Program, an applicable beneficiary shall agree to receive opioid use disorder treatment services from a participant. Participation under the Program shall not affect coverage of or payment for any other item or service under this title for the applicable beneficiary.

(4) BENEFICIARY ACCESS TO SERVICES.—Nothing in this section shall be construed as encouraging providers to limit applicable beneficiary access to services covered under this title and applicable beneficiaries shall not be required to relinquish access to any benefit under this title as a condition of receiving services from a participant in the Program.

(e) PAYMENTS.—

(1) PER APPLICABLE BENEFICIARY PER MONTH CARE MANAGEMENT FEE.—

(A) IN GENERAL.—The Secretary shall establish a schedule of per applicable beneficiary per month care management fees. Such a per applicable beneficiary per month care management fee shall be paid to a participant in addition to any other amount otherwise payable under this title to the health care practitioners in the participant's opioid use disorder care team or, if applicable, to the participant. A participant may use such per applicable beneficiary per month care management fee to deliver additional services to applicable beneficiaries, including services not otherwise eligible for payment under this title.

(B) PAYMENT AMOUNTS.—In carrying out subparagraph (A), the Secretary shall—

(i) (consider payments otherwise payable under this title for opioid use disorder treatment services and the needs of applicable beneficiaries;

(ii) pay a higher per applicable beneficiary per month care management fee for an applicable beneficiary who receives more intensive treatment services from a participant and for whom those services are appropriate based on clinical guidelines for opioid use disorder care;

(iii) pay a higher per applicable beneficiary per month care management fee for the month in which the applicable beneficiary begins treatment with a participant than in subsequent months, to reflect the greater time and costs required for the planning and initiation of treatment, as compared to maintenance of treatment;

(iv) pay higher per applicable beneficiary per month care management fees for participants that have established opioid use disorder care teams that include an addiction specialist (as defined in subsection (c)(3)(B)); and

(v) take into account whether a participant's opioid use disorder care team refers applicable beneficiaries to other suppliers or providers for any opioid use disorder treatment services.

(2) INCENTIVE PAYMENTS.—

(A) IN GENERAL.—Under the Program, the Secretary shall establish a performance-based incentive payment, which shall be paid (using a methodology established and at a time determined appropriate by the Secretary) to participants based on the performance of participants with respect to criteria, as determined appropriate by the Secretary, in accordance with subparagraph (B).

(B) CRITERIA.—

(i) IN GENERAL.—Criteria described in subparagraph (A) may include consideration of the following:

(I) Patient engagement and retention in treatment.

(II) Evidence-based medication-assisted treatment.

(III) Other criteria established by the Secretary.

REQUIRED CONSULTATION AND CONSIDERATION.— In determining criteria described in subparagraph (A), the Secretary shall—

(I) consult with stakeholders, including clinicians in the primary care community and in the field of addiction medicine; and

(II) consider existing clinical guidelines for the treatment of opioid use disorders.

(C) SUBMISSION OF DATA.—Each participant shall submit to the Secretary, in such form, manner, and frequency specified by the Secretary, data with respect to such criteria described in subparagraph (A) and such other information as the Secretary determines appropriate to evaluate and monitor the effectiveness of the Program, to determine the performance of the participants for purposes of the incentive payment under subparagraph (A), and to ensure the participants meet minimum criteria for program participation described in subsection (c)(2)(B)(ii).

(3) NON-DUPLICATION OF PAYMENTS.—In the case if an applicable beneficiary receiving services supported by the Program from more than one participant during any one calendar month, or from a participant and a provider who is not a participant during any one calendar month, the Secretary shall adjust (such as pro-rate) payment under paragraph (1) and any payment under paragraph (2) to each such participant, with respect to such applicable beneficiary and month to avoid any duplication of payment.

(f) MULTIPAYER STRATEGY.—In carrying out the Program, the Secretary shall encourage other payers to provide similar payments and to use similar criteria as applied under the Program under subsection (e)(2)(C). The Secretary may enter into a memorandum of understanding with other payers to align the methodology for payment provided by such a payer related to opioid use disorder treatment services with such methodology for payment under the Program.

(g) EVALUATION.—

(1) IN GENERAL.—The Secretary shall conduct an intermediate and final evaluation of the program. Each such evaluation shall determine the extent to which each of the purposes described in subsection (b) have been accomplished under the Program.

(2) REPORTS.—The Secretary shall submit to the Secretary and Congress—

(A) a report with respect to the intermediate evaluation under paragraph (1) not later than 3 years after the date of the implementation of the Program; and

(B) a report with respect to the final evaluation under paragraph (1) not later than 6 years after such date.

(h) FUNDING.—

(1) ADMINISTRATIVE FUNDING.—For the purposes of implementing, administering, and carrying out the Program (other than for purposes described in paragraph (2)), the Secretary shall provide for the transfer from the Federal Supplementary Medical Insurance Trust Fund under section 1841 of $5,000,000 to the Centers for Medicare & Medicaid Services Program Management Account.

(2) CARE MANAGEMENT FEES AND INCENTIVES.—For the purposes of making payments under subsection (e), the Secretary shall provide for the transfer from the Federal Supplementary Medical Insurance Trust Fund under section 1841 of $10,000,000 for each of fiscal years 2021 through 2025.

(3) AVAILABILITY.—Amounts transferred under this subsection for a fiscal year shall be available until expended.

(i) WAIVERS.—The Secretary may waive any provision of this title as may be necessary to carry out the Program under this section.

## Exchange of Letters with Additional Committees of Referral

GREG WALDEN, OREGON
CHAIRMAN

FRANK PALLONE, JR., NEW JERSEY
RANKING MEMBER

ONE HUNDRED FIFTEENTH CONGRESS

**Congress of the United States**

**House of Representatives**

COMMITTEE ON ENERGY AND COMMERCE
2125 RAYBURN HOUSE OFFICE BUILDING
WASHINGTON, DC 20515–6115
Majority (202) 225-2927
Minority (202) 225-3641

June 7, 2018

The Honorable Kevin Brady
Chairman
Committee on Ways and Means
1102 Longworth House Office Building
Washington, DC 20515

Dear Chairman Brady:

On May 9 and 17, 2018, the Committee on Energy and Commerce ordered favorably reported over 50 bills to address the opioid epidemic facing communities across our nation. Several of the bills were also referred to the Committee on Ways and Means.

I ask that the Committee on Ways and Means not insist on its referral of the following bills so that they may be scheduled for consideration by the Majority Leader:

- **H.R. 1925**, At-Risk Youth Medicaid Protection Act of 2017;
- **H.R. 3331**, To amend title XI of the Social Security Act to promote testing of incentive payments for behavioral health providers for adoption and use of certified electronic health record technology;
- **H.R. 3528**, Every Prescription Conveyed Securely Act;
- **H.R. 4841**, Standardizing Electronic Prior Authorization for Safe Prescribing Act of 2018;
- **H.R. 5582**, Abuse Deterrent Access Act of 2018;
- **H.R. 5590**, Opioid Addiction Action Plan Act;
- **H.R. 5603**, Access to Telehealth Services for Opioid Use Disorder;

The Honorable Kevin Brady
Page 2

- **H.R. 5605**, Advancing High Quality Treatment for Opioid Use Disorders in Medicare Act;
- **H.R. 5675**, To amend title XVIII of the Social Security Act to require prescription drug plan sponsors under the Medicare program to establish drug management programs for at-risk beneficiaries;
- **H.R. 5684**, Protecting Seniors from Opioid Abuse Act;
- **H.R. 5685**, Medicare Opioid Safety Education Act;
- **H.R. 5686**, Medicare Clear Health Options in Care for Enrollees (CHOICE) Act;
- **H.R. 5715**, Strengthening Partnerships to Prevent Opioid Abuse Act;
- **H.R. 5716**, Commit to Opioid Medical Prescriber Accountability and Safety for Seniors (COMPASS) Act;
- **H.R. 5796**, Responsible Education Achieves Care and Healthy Outcomes for Users' Treatment (REACH OUT) Act of 2018;
- **H.R. 5798**, Opioid Screening and Chronic Pain Management Alternatives for Seniors Act;
- **H.R. 5804**, Post-Surgical Injections as an Opioid Alternative Act; and
- **H.R. 5809**, Postoperative Opioid Prevention Act of 2018.

This concession in no way affects your jurisdiction over the subject matter of these bills, and it will not serve as precedent for future referrals. In addition, should a conference on the bills be necessary, I would support your request to have the Committee on Ways and Means on the conference committee. Finally, I would be pleased to include this letter and your response in the bill reports and the Congressional Record.

Thank you for your consideration of my request and for the extraordinary cooperation shown by you and your staff over matters of shared jurisdiction. I look forward to further opportunities to work with you this Congress.

Sincerely,

Greg Walden
Chairman

Congress of the United States
U.S. House of Representatives
COMMITTEE ON WAYS AND MEANS
1102 LONGWORTH HOUSE OFFICE BUILDING
(202) 225-3625
Washington, DC 20515-0348
http://waysandmeans.house.gov

June 8, 2018

The Honorable Greg Walden
Chairman
Committee on Energy and Commerce
2125 Rayburn House Office Building
Washington, DC 20515

Dear Chairman Walden,

Thank you for your letter concerning several bills favorably reported out of the Committee on Energy and Commerce to address the opioid epidemic and which the Committee on Ways and Means was granted an additional referral.

As a result of your having consulted with us on provisions within these bills that fall within the Rule X jurisdiction of the Committee on Ways and Means, I agree to waive formal consideration of the following bills so that they may move expeditiously to the floor:

- **H.R. 1925**, At-Risk Youth Medicaid Protection Act of 2017;
- **H.R. 3331**, To amend title XI of the Social Security Act to promote testing of incentive payments for behavioral health providers for adoption and use of certified electronic health record technology;
- **H.R. 3528**, Every Prescription Conveyed Securely Act;
- **H.R. 4841**, Standardizing Electronic Prior Authorization for Safe Prescribing Act of 2018;
- **H.R. 5582**, Abuse Deterrent Access Act of 2018;
- **H.R. 5590**, Opioid Addiction Action Plan Act;
- **H.R. 5603**, Access to Telehealth Services for Opioid Use Disorder;
- **H.R. 5605**, Advancing High Quality Treatment for Opioid Use Disorders in Medicare Act;

- **H.R. 5675,** To amend title XVIII of the Social Security Act to require prescription drug plan sponsors under the Medicare program to establish drug management programs for at-risk beneficiaries;
- **H.R. 5684,** Protecting Seniors from Opioid Abuse Act;
- **H.R. 5685,** Medicare Opioid Safety Education Act;
- **H.R. 5686,** Medicare Clear Health Options in Care for Enrollees (CHOICE) Act;
- **H.R. 5715,** Strengthening Partnerships to Prevent Opioid Abuse Act;
- **H.R. 5716,** Commit to Opioid Medical Prescriber Accountability and Safety for Seniors (COMPASS) Act;
- **H.R. 5796,** Responsible Education Achieves Care and Healthy Outcomes for Users' Treatment (REACH OUT) Act of 2018;
- **H.R. 5798,** Opioid Screening and Chronic Pain Management Alternatives for Seniors Act;
- **H.R. 5804,** Post-Surgical Injections as an Opioid Alternative Act; and
- **H.R. 5809,** Postoperative Opioid Prevention Act of 2018.

The Committee on Ways and Means takes this action with the mutual understanding that we do not waive any jurisdiction over the subject matter contained in this or similar legislation, and the Committee will be appropriately consulted and involved as the bill or similar legislation moves forward so that we may address any remaining issues that fall within our jurisdiction. The Committee also reserves the right to seek appointment of an appropriate number of conferees to any House-Senate conference involving this or similar legislation and requests your support for such a request.

Finally, I would appreciate your commitment to include this exchange of letters in the bill reports and the Congressional Record.

Sincerely,

Kevin Brady
Chairman

cc: The Honorable Paul Ryan, Speaker
The Honorable Richard E. Neal
The Honorable Frank Pallone
Thomas J. Wickham, Jr., Parliamentarian

In: Opioid Use and Misuse …
Editor: Tom Freitag
ISBN: 978-1-53616-858-7


*Chapter 3*

# STRENGTHENING PARTNERSHIPS TO PREVENT OPIOID ABUSE ACT*

***Committee on Energy and Commerce***

Mr. Walden, from the Committee on Energy and Commerce, submitted the following report [To accompany H.R. 5715] [Including cost estimate of the Congressional Budget Office]

The Committee on Energy and Commerce, to whom was referred the bill (H.R. 5715) to amend title XVIII of the Social Security Act to provide for certain program integrity transparency measures under Medicare parts C and D, having considered the same, report favorably thereon with an amendment and recommend that the bill as amended do pass.

The amendment is as follows:

Strike all after the enacting clause and insert the following:

* This is an edited, reformatted and augmented version of House of Representatives 115th Congress, 2d Session, REPT. 115–737, Part 1, dated June 12, 2018.

## SECTION 1. SHORT TITLE

This Act may be cited as the "Strengthening Partnerships to Prevent Opioid Abuse Act".

## SEC. 2. PROGRAM INTEGRITY TRANSPARENCY MEASURES UNDER MEDICARE PARTS C AND D

IN GENERAL.—Section 1859 of the Social Security Act (42 U.S.C. 1395w–28) is amended by adding at the end the following new subsection:

"(i) PROGRAM INTEGRITY TRANSPARENCY MEASURES.— "(1) PROGRAM INTEGRITY PORTAL.—

"(A) IN GENERAL.—Not later than two years after the date of the enactment of this subsection, the Secretary shall, after consultation with stakeholders, establish a secure Internet website portal (or other successor technology) that would allow a secure path for communication between the Secretary, MA plans under this part, prescription drug plans under part D, and an eligible entity with a contract under section 1893 (such as a Medi care drug integrity contractor or an entity responsible for carrying out pro gram integrity activities under this part and part D) for the purpose of ena bling through such portal (or other successor technology)—

"(i) the referral by such plans of substantiated fraud, waste, and abuse for initiating or assisting investigations conducted by the eligible entity; and

"(ii) data sharing among such MA plans, prescription drug plans, and the Secretary.

"(B) REQUIRED USES OF PORTAL.—The Secretary shall disseminate the following information to MA plans under this part and prescription drug plans under part D through the secure Internet website portal (or other successor technology) established under subparagraph (A):

"(i) Providers of services and suppliers that have been referred pursuant to subparagraph (A)(i) during the previous 12-month period.

"(ii) Providers of services and suppliers who are the subject of an active exclusion under section 1128 or who are subject to a suspension of payment under this title pursuant to section 1862(o) or otherwise.

"(iii) Providers of services and suppliers who are the subject of an active revocation of participation under this title, including for not satis fying conditions of participation.

"(iv) In the case of such a plan that makes a referral under subpara graph (A)(i) through the portal (or other successor technology) with re spect to activities of substantiated fraud, waste, or abuse of a provider of services or supplier, if such provider or supplier has been the subject of an administrative action under this title or title XI with respect to similar activities, a notification to such plan of such action so taken. "(C) RULEMAKING.—For purposes of this paragraph, the Secretary shall, through rulemaking, specify what constitutes substantiated fraud, waste, and abuse, using guidance such as what is provided in the Medicare Program Integrity Manual 4.7.1. In carrying out the previous sentence, for purposes of this paragraph, a fraud hotline tip (as defined by the Secretary) without further evidence shall not be treated as sufficient evidence for substantiated fraud, waste, or abuse.

"(D) HIPAA COMPLIANT INFORMATION ONLY.—For purposes of this subsection, communications may only occur if the communications are permitted under the Federal regulations (concerning the privacy of individually identifiable health information) promulgated under section 264(c) of the Health Insurance Portability and Accountability Act of 1996.

"(2) QUARTERLY REPORTS.—Beginning two years after the date of enactment of this subsection, the Secretary shall make available to MA plans under this part and prescription drug plans under part D in a timely manner (but no less frequently than quarterly) and using information submitted to an entity described in paragraph (1) through the portal (or other successor technology) described in such paragraph or pursuant to section 1893, information on fraud, waste, and abuse schemes and trends in identifying suspicious activity. Information included in each such report shall—

"(A) include administrative actions, pertinent information related to opioid overprescribing, and other data determined appropriate by the Sec retary in consultation with stakeholders; and

"(B) be anonymized information submitted by plans without identifying the source of such information.

"(3) CLARIFICATION.—Nothing in this subsection shall be construed as precluding or otherwise affecting referrals described in subparagraph (A) that may otherwise be made to law enforcement entities or to the Secretary."

CONTRACT REQUIREMENT TO COMMUNICATE PLAN CORRECTIVE ACTIONS AGAINST OPIOIDS OVER-PRESCRIBERS.—Section 1857(e) of the Social Security Act (42

U.S.C. 1395w–27(e)) is amended by adding at the end the following new paragraph: "(5) COMMUNICATING PLAN CORRECTIVE CTIONS AGAINST OPIOIDS OVER-PRESCRIBERS.—

"(A) IN GENERAL.—Beginning with plan years beginning on or after January 1, 2021, a contract under this section with an MA organization shall require the organization to submit to the Secretary, through the process established under subparagraph (B), information on the investigations and other actions taken by such plans related to providers of services who prescribe a high volume of opioids.

"(B) PROCESS.—Not later than January 1, 2021, the Secretary shall, in consultation with stakeholders, establish a process under which MA plans and prescription drug plans shall submit to the Secretary information described in subparagraph (A).

"(C) REGULATIONS.—For purposes of this paragraph, including as applied under section 1860D–12(b)(3)(D), the Secretary shall, pursuant to rulemaking—

"(i) specify a definition for the term 'high volume of opioids' and a method for determining if a provider of services prescribes such a high volume; and

"(ii) establish the process described in subparagraph (B) and the types of information that shall be submitted through such process."

REFERENCE UNDER PART D TO PROGRAM INTEGRITY TRANSPARENCY MEASURES.—Section 1860D–4 of the Social Security Act (42 U.S.C. 1395w–104) is amended by adding at the end the following new subsection:

"(m) PROGRAM INTEGRITY TRANSPARENCY MEASURES.—For program integrity transparency measures applied with respect to prescription drug plan and MA plans, see section 1859(i)."

## PURPOSE AND SUMMARY

H.R. 5715, Strengthening Partnerships to Prevent Opioid Abuse Act, was introduced on May 9, 2018, by Rep. James Renacci (R– OH), Rep. Terri Sewell (D–AL), Rep. Brett Guthrie (R–KY), and Rep. Scott Peters (D–CA) to help facilitate communication among Medicare Advantage (MA) organizations, Part D plan sponsors, and the Centers for Medicare and Medicaid Services (CMS) relating to substantiated fraud, waste, and abuse investigations.

## BACKGROUND AND NEED FOR LEGISLATION

The Medicare program serves as the healthcare coverage provider to over 58 million beneficiaries. This number is projected to rise to over 80 million by 2030. In serving the over age 65 population, Medicare accounts for a large share of total opioid prescriptions. In 2016, one out of every three beneficiaries was prescribed an opioid through Medicare Part D. In total, this equates to almost 80 million prescriptions and $4 billion in Medicare Part D spending. While many Medicare beneficiaries with serious pain-related conditions are being properly prescribed opioids, there is mounting evidence of opioid misuse in the Medicare system. As more seniors and individuals with disabilities come into the program, the chal lenges of fraud, misuse, and abuse will only increase.

This bill seeks to strengthen program integrity by improving communication among plan sponsors and CMS to better identify potential fraud, waste, and abuse.

## COMMITTEE ACTION

On April 11 and 12, 2018, the Subcommittee on Health held a hearing entitled "Combating the Opioid Crisis: Improving the Ability of Medicare and Medicaid to Provide Care for Patients" to review legislation related to the opioid epidemic. The Subcommittee received testimony from:

- Kimberly Brandt, Principal Deputy Administrator for Operations, Centers for Medicare and Medicaid Services, U.S. Department of Health and Human Services;
- Michael Botticelli, Executive Director, Grayken Center for Addiction, Boston Medical Center;
- Toby Douglas, Senior Vice President, Medicaid Solutions, Centene Corporation;
- David Guth, CEO, Centerstone;
- John Kravitz, CIO, Geisinger Health System; and,
- Sam Srivastava, CEO, Magellan Health.

On April 25, 2018, the Subcommittee on Health met in open markup session and forwarded a discussion draft, entitled "CMS/ Plan Sharing," without amendment, to the full Committee by a voice vote. On May 17, 2018, the full Committee on Energy and Commerce met in open markup session and ordered H.R. 5715, as amended, favorable reported to the House by a voice vote. H.R. 5715 was similar to the discussion draft forwarded by the Subcommittee.

## COMMITTEE VOTES

Clause 3(b) of rule XIII requires the Committee to list the record votes on the motion to report legislation and amendments thereto. There were no record votes taken in connection with ordering H.R. 5715 reported.

## OVERSIGHT FINDINGS AND RECOMMENDATIONS

Pursuant to clause 2(b)(1) of rule X and clause 3(c)(1) of rule XIII, the Committee held a hearing and made findings that are reflected in this report.

## NEW BUDGET AUTHORITY, ENTITLEMENT AUTHORITY, AND TAX EXPENDITURES

Pursuant to clause 3(c)(2) of rule XIII, the Committee finds that H.R. 5715 would result in no new or increased budget authority, entitlement authority, or tax expenditures or revenues.

## CONGRESSIONAL BUDGET OFFICE ESTIMATE

Pursuant to clause 3(c)(3) of rule XIII, the following is the cost estimate provided by the Congressional Budget Office pursuant to section 402 of the Congressional Budget Act of 1974:

U.S. Congress, Congressional Budget Office,
Washington, DC, June 6, 2018.
Hon. GREG WALDEN,

Chairman, Committee on Energy and Commerce, House of Representatives, Washington, DC.

DEAR MR. CHAIRMAN: The Congressional Budget Office has pre pared the enclosed document with cost estimates for the opioid-related legislation ordered to be reported on May 9 and May 17, 2018.

If you wish further details on this estimate, we will be pleased to provide them. The CBO staff contacts are Tom Bradley and Chad Chirico.

Sincerely,

Mark P. Hadley
(For Keith Hall, Director)

## Opioid Legislation

Summary: On May 9 and May 17, 2018, the House Committee on Energy and Commerce ordered 59 bills to be reported related to the nation's response to the opioid epidemic. Generally, the bills would:

- Provide grants to facilities and providers that treat people with substance use disorders,
- Direct various agencies within the Department of Health and Human Services (HHS) to explore nonopioid approaches to treating pain and to educate providers about those alternatives,
- Modify requirements under Medicaid and Medicare for prescribing controlled substances,
- Expand Medicaid coverage for substance abuse treatment, and
- Direct the Food and Drug Administration (FDA) to modify its oversight of opioid drugs and other medications that are used to manage pain.

Because of the large number of related bills ordered reported by the Committee, CBO is publishing a single comprehensive document that includes estimates for each piece of legislation.

CBO estimates that enacting 20 of the bills would affect direct spending, and 2 of the bills would affect revenues; therefore, payas-you-go procedures apply for those bills.

CBO estimates that enacting H.R. 4998, the Health Insurance for Former Foster Youth Act, would increase net direct spending by more than $2.5 billion and on-budget deficits by more than $5 billion in at least one of the four consecutive 10-year periods beginning in 2029. None of the remaining 58 bills included in this estimate would increase net direct spending by more than $2.5 billion or on-budget deficits by more than $5 billion in any of the four consecutive 10-year periods beginning in 2029.

One of the bills reviewed for this document, H.R. 5795, would impose both intergovernmental and private-sector mandates as defined in the Unfunded Mandates Reform Act (UMRA). CBO estimates that the costs of those mandates on public and private entities would fall below the thresholds in UMRA ($80 million and $160 million, respectively, in 2018, adjusted annually for inflation). Five bills, H.R. 5228, H.R. 5333, H.R. 5554, H.R. 5687, and H.R.

5811, would impose private-sector mandates as defined in UMRA. CBO estimates that the costs of the mandates in three of the bills (H.R. 5333, H.R. 5554, and H.R. 5811) would not exceed the UMRA threshold for private entities. Because CBO is uncertain how federal agencies would implement new authority granted in the other two bills, H.R. 5228 and H.R. 5687, CBO cannot determine whether the costs of those mandates would exceed the UMRA threshold.

Estimated cost to the Federal Government: The estimates in this document do not include the effects of interactions among the bills. If all 59 bills were combined and enacted as one piece of legislation, the budgetary effects would be different from the sum of the estimates in this document, although CBO expects that any such differences would be small. The costs of this legislation fall within budget functions 550 (health), 570 (Medicare), 750 (administration of justice), and 800 (general government).

Basis of estimate: For this estimate, CBO assumes that all of the legislation will be enacted late in 2018 and that authorized and estimated amounts will be appropriated each year. Outlays for discretionary programs are estimated based on historical spending patterns for similar programs.

## Uncertainty

CBO aims to produce estimates that generally reflect the middle of a range of the most likely budgetary outcomes that would result if the legislation was enacted. Because data on the utilization of mental health and substance abuse treatment under Medicaid and Medicare is scarce, CBO cannot precisely predict how patients or providers would respond to some policy changes or what budgetary effects would result. In addition, several of the bills would give the Department of Health and Human Services (HHS) considerable latitude in designing and implementing policies. Budgetary effects could differ from those provided in CBO's analyses depending on those decisions.

## Direct Spending and Revenues

Table 1 lists the 22 bills of the 59 ordered to be reported that would affect direct spending or revenues.

Legislation Primarily Affecting Medicaid. The following nine bills would affect direct spending for the Medicaid program.

## Table 1. Estimated changes in mandatory spending and revenues

| | By fiscal year, in millions of dollars— | | | | | | | | | | | |
|---|---|---|---|---|---|---|---|---|---|---|---|---|
| | **2018** | **2019** | **2020** | **2021** | **2022** | **2023** | **2024** | **2025** | **2026** | **2027** | **2028** | **2019-2023** | **2019-2028** |
| | Increases Or Decreases (-) In Direct Spending | | | | | | | | | | | | |
| Legislation Primarily Affecting Medicaid: | | | | | | | | | | | | | |
| H.R. 1925, At-Risk Youth Medicaid Protection Act of 2017 | 0 | * | 5 | 5 | 5 | 10 | 10 | 10 | 10 | 10 | 10 | 25 | 75 |
| H.R. 4998, Health Insurance for Former Foster Youth Act | 0 | 0 | 0 | 0 | 0 | * | 10 | 21 | 33 | 46 | 61 | * | 171 |
| H.R. 5477, Rural Development of Opioid Capacity Services Act | 0 | 13 | 35 | 58 | 68 | 83 | 27 | 9 | 3 | 3 | 3 | 256 | 301 |
| H.R. 5583, a bill to amend title XI of the Social Security Act to require States to annually report on certain adult health quality measures, and for other purposes | 0 | * | * | * | * | * | * | * | * | * | * | * | * |
| H.R. 5797, IMD CARE Act | 0 | 38 | 158 | 251 | 265 | 279 | 0 | 0 | 0 | 0 | 0 | 991 | 991 |
| H.R. 5799, Medicaid DRUG Improvement Act[a] | 0 | * | * | 1 | 1 | 1 | 1 | 1 | 1 | 1 | 1 | 2 | 5 |
| H.R. 5801, Medicaid Providers Are Required To Note Experiences in Record Systems to Help In-Need Patients (PARTNERSHIP) Act[a] | 0 | * | * | * | * | * | * | * | * | * | * | * | * |
| H.R. 5808, Medicaid Pharmaceutical Home Act of 2018[a] | 0 | * | -1 | -1 | -1 | -1 | -2 | -2 | -2 | -2 | -2 | -4 | -13 |
| H.R. 5810, Medicaid Health HOME Act | 0 | 94 | 58 | 62 | 56 | 52 | 48 | 43 | 38 | 32 | 25 | 323 | 509 |
| Legislation Primarily Affecting Medicare: | | | | | | | | | | | | | |
| H.R. 3528, Every Prescription Conveyed Securely Act | 0 | 0 | 0 | -24 | -35 | -33 | -30 | -33 | -32 | -31 | -32 | -92 | -250 |
| H.R. 4841, Standardizing Electronic Prior Authorization for Safe Prescribing Act of 2018 | 0 | 0 | * | * | * | * | * | * | * | * | * | * | * |
| H.R. 5603, Access to Telehealth Services for Opioid Use Disorders Act | 0 | 2 | * | * | * | 1 | 1 | 1 | 2 | 2 | 2 | 3 | 11 |

**Table 1. (Continued)**

| | By fiscal year, in millions of dollars— | | | | | | | | | | | | |
|---|---|---|---|---|---|---|---|---|---|---|---|---|---|
| | 2018 | 2019 | 2020 | 2021 | 2022 | 2023 | 2024 | 2025 | 2026 | 2027 | 2028 | 2019-2023 | 2019-2028 |
| H.R. 5605, Advancing High Quality Treatment for Opioid Use Disorders in Medicare Act | 0 | 0 | 0 | 15 | 26 | 24 | 23 | 23 | 10 | 1 | * | 65 | 122 |
| H.R. 5675, a bill to amend title XVIII of the Social Security Act to require prescription drug plan sponsors under the Medicare program to establish drug management programs for at-risk beneficiaries | 0 | 0 | 0 | -6 | -7 | -7 | -7 | -8 | -9 | -9 | -11 | -20 | -64 |
| H.R. 5684, Protecting Seniors From Opioid Abuse Act | 0 | 0 | * | * | * | * | * | * | * | * | * | * | * |
| H.R. 5796, Responsible Education Achieves Care and Healthy Outcomes for Users' Treatment Act of 2018 | 0 | 10 | 25 | 50 | 10 | 5 | 0 | 0 | 0 | 0 | 0 | 100 | 100 |
| H.R. 5798, Opioid Screening and Chronic Pain Management Alternatives for Seniors Act | 0 | 0 | * | 1 | 1 | 1 | 1 | 1 | 1 | 1 | 1 | 2 | 5 |
| H.R. 5804, Post-Surgical Injections as an Opioid Alternative Act[a] | 0 | 0 | 25 | 30 | 25 | 20 | 10 | 5 | 0 | 0 | 0 | 100 | 115 |
| H.R. 5809, Postoperative Opioid Prevention Act of 2018 | 0 | 0 | 0 | 0 | 10 | 15 | 20 | 25 | 30 | 35 | 45 | 25 | 180 |
| Legislation Primarily Affecting the Food and Drug Administration: | | | | | | | | | | | | | |
| H.R. 5333, Over-the-Counter Monograph Safety, Innovation, and Reform Act of 2018[a] | 0 | 0 | * | * | * | * | * | * | * | * | * | * | * |
| H.R. 5333, Over-the-Counter Monograph Safety, Innovation, and Reform Act of 2018[a] | 0 | * | * | * | * | * | * | * | * | * | * | * | * |

Annual amounts may not sum to totals because of rounding. * = between -$500,000 and $500,000. Budget authority is equivalent to outlays.

[a] This bill also would affect spending subject to appropriation.

[b] One additional bill, H.R. 5228, the Stop Counterfeit Drugs by Regulating and Enhancing Enforcement Now Act, would have a negligible effect on revenues.

*H.R. 1925, the At-Risk Youth Medicaid Protection Act of 2017,* would require states to suspend, rather than terminate, Medicaid eligibility for juvenile enrollees (generally under 21 years of age) who become inmates of public correctional institutions. States also would have to redetermine those enrollees' Medicaid eligibility before their release and restore their coverage upon release if they qualify for the program. States would be required to process Medicaid applications submitted by or on behalf of juveniles in public correctional institutions who were not enrolled in Medicaid before becoming inmates and ensure that Medicaid coverage is provided when they are released if they are found to be eligible. On the basis of an analysis of juvenile incarceration trends and of the per enrollee spending for Medicaid foster care children, who have a similar health profile to incarcerated juveniles, CBO estimates that implementing the bill would cost $75 million over the 2019–2028 period.

*H.R. 4998, the Health Insurance for Former Foster Youth Act,* would require states to provide Medicaid coverage to adults up to age 25 who had aged out of foster care in any state. Under current law, such coverage is mandatory only if the former foster care youth has aged out in the state in which the individual applies for coverage. The policy also would apply to former foster children who had been in foster care upon turning 14 years of age but subsequently left foster care to enter into a legal guardianship with a kinship caregiver. The provisions would take effect respect for fos ter youth who turn 18 on or after January 1, 2023. On the basis of spending for Medicaid foster care children and data from the Census Bureau regarding annual migration rates between states, CBO estimates that implementing the bill would cost $171 million over the 2019–2028 period.

*H.R. 5477, the Rural Development of Opioid Capacity Services Act,* would direct the Secretary of HHS to conduct a five-year demonstration to increase the number and ability of providers participating in Medicaid to provide treatment for substance use disorders. On the basis of an analysis of federal and state spending for treatment of substance use disorders and the prevalence of such disorders, CBO estimates that enacting the bill would increase direct spending by $301 million over the 2019–2028 period.

*H.R. 5583, a bill to amend title XI of the Social Security Act to require States to annually report on certain adult health quality measures, and for other purposes,* would require states to include behavioral health indicators in their annual reports on the quality of care under Medicaid. Although the bill would add a requirement for states, CBO estimates that its enactment would not have a significant budgetary effect because most states have systems in place for reporting such measures to the federal government.

*H.R. 5797, the IMD CARE Act,* would expand Medicaid coverage for people with opioid use disorder who are in institutions for mental disease (IMDs) for up to 30 days per year. Under a current-law policy known as the IMD exclusion, the federal government generally does not make matching payments to state Medicaid programs for most services provided by IMDs to adults between the ages of 21 and 64. Recent administrative changes have made federal financing for IMDs available in limited circumstances, but the statutory prohibition remains in place. CBO analyzed several data sets, primarily those collected by the Substance Abuse and Mental Health Services Administration (SAMHSA), to estimate current federal spending under Medicaid for IMD services and to estimate spending under H.R. 5797. Using that analysis, CBO estimates that enacting H.R. 5797 would increase direct spending by $991 million over the 2019–2028 period.

*H.R. 5799, the Medicaid DRUG Improvement Act,* would require state Medicaid programs to implement additional reviews of opioid prescriptions, monitor concurrent prescribing of opioids and certain other drugs, and monitor use of antipsychotic drugs by children. CBO estimates that the bill would increase direct spending by $5 million over 2019–2028 period to cover the administrative costs of complying with those requirements. On the basis of stakeholder feedback, CBO expects that the bill would not have a significant effect on Medicaid spending for prescription drugs because many of the bill's requirements would duplicate current efforts to curb opioid and antipsychotic drug use. (If enacted, H.R. 5799 also would affect spending subject to appropriation; CBO has not completed an estimate of that amount).

*H.R. 5801, the Medicaid Providers Are Required To Note Experiences in Record Systems to Help-In-Need Patients (PARTNERSHIP) Act,* would require providers who are permitted to prescribe controlled substances and who participate in Medicaid to query prescription drug monitoring programs (PDMPs) before prescribing controlled substances to Medicaid patients. PDMPs are statewide electronic databases that collect data on controlled substances dispensed in the state. The bill also would require PDMPs to comply with certain data and system criteria, and it would provide additional federal matching funds to certain states to help cover administrative costs. On the basis of a literature review and stakeholder feedback, CBO estimates that the net budgetary effect of enacting H.R. 5801 would be insignificant. Costs for states to come into compliance with the systems and administrative requirements would be roughly offset by savings from small reductions in the number of controlled substances paid for by Medicaid under the proposal. (If enacted, H.R. 5801 also would affect spending subject to appropriation; CBO has not completed an estimate of that amount).

*H.R. 5808, the Medicaid Pharmaceutical Home Act of 2018,* would require state Medicaid programs to operate pharmacy programs that would identify people at high risk of abusing controlled substances and require those patients to use a limited number of providers and pharmacies. Although nearly all state Medicaid programs currently meet such a requirement, a small number of highrisk Medicaid beneficiaries are not now monitored. Based on an analysis of information about similar state and federal programs, CBO estimates that net Medicaid spending under the bill would decrease by $13 million over the 2019–2028 period. That amount represents a small increase in administrative costs and a small reduction in the number of controlled substances paid for by Medicaid under the proposal. (If enacted, H.R. 5808 also would affect spending subject to appropriation; CBO has not completed an estimate of that amount).

*H.R. 5810, the Medicaid Health HOME Act,* would allow states to receive six months of enhanced federal Medicaid funding for programs that coordinate care for people with substance use disorders. Based on enrollment and spending data from states that currently participate in Medicaid's Health Homes program, CBO estimates that the expansion would cost approximately $469 million over the 2019–2028 period. The bill also would require states to cover all FDA-approved drugs used in medication-assisted treatment for five years, although states could seek a waiver from that requirement. (Medication-assisted treatment combines behavioral therapy and pharmaceutical treatment for substance use disorders). Under current law, states already cover most FDA-approved drugs used in such programs in some capacity, although a few exclude methadone dispensed by opioid treatment programs. CBO estimates that a small share of those states would begin to cover methadone if this bill was enacted at a federal cost of about $39 million over the 2019–2028 period. In sum, CBO estimates that the enacting H.R. 5810 would increase direct spending by $509 million over the 2019–2028 period.

Legislation Primarily Affecting Medicare. The following ten bills would affect direct spending for the Medicare program.

*H.R. 3528, the Every Prescription Conveyed Securely Act,* would require prescriptions for controlled substances covered under Medicare Part D to be transmitted electronically, starting on January 1, 2021. Based on CBO's analysis of prescription drug spending, spending for controlled substances is a small share of total drug spending. CBO also assumes a small share of those prescriptions would not be filled because they are not converted to an electronic format. Therefore, CBO expects that enacting H.R. 3528 would reduce the number of prescriptions filled and estimates that Medicare spending would be reduced by $250 million over the 2019–2028 period.

*H.R. 4841, the Standardizing Electronic Prior Authorization for Safe Prescribing Act of 2018,* would require health care professionals to submit prior authorization requests electronically, starting on January 1, 2021, for drugs covered under Medicare Part D. Taking into account that many prescribers already use electronic methods to submit such requests, CBO estimates that enacting H.R. 4841 would not significantly affect direct spending for Part D.

*H.R. 5603, the Access to Telehealth Services for Opioid Use Dis orders Act,* would permit the Secretary of HHS to lift current geographic and other restrictions on coverage of telehealth services under Medicare for treatment of substance use disorders or co-occurring mental health disorders. Under the bill, the Secretary of HHS would be directed to encourage other payers to coordinate payments for opioid use disorder treatments and to evaluate the extent to which the demonstration reduces hospitalizations, increases the use of medication-assisted treatments, and improves the health outcomes of individuals with opioid use disorders during and after the demonstration. Based on current use of Medicare telehealth services for treatment of substance use disorders, CBO estimates that expanding that coverage would increase direct spending by $11 million over the 2019–2028 period.

*H.R. 5605, the Advancing High Quality Treatment* for Opioid Use Disorders in Medicare Act, would establish a five-year demonstration program to increase access to treatment for opioid use disorder. The demonstration would provide incentive payments and funding for care management services based on criteria such as patient engagement, use of evidence-based treatments, and treatment length and intensity. Under the bill, the Secretary of HHS would be directed to encourage other payers to coordinate payments for opioid use disorder treatments and to evaluate the extent to which the demonstration reduces hospitalizations, increases the use of medication-assisted treatments, and improves the health outcomes of individuals with opioid use disorders during and after the demonstration. Based on historical utilization of opioid use disorder treatments and projected spending on incentive payments and care management fees, CBO estimates that increased use of treatment services and the demonstration's incentive payments would increase direct spending by $122 million over the 2019–2028 period.

*H.R. 5675, a bill to amend title XVIII of the Social Security Act to require prescription drug plan sponsors under the Medicare program to establish drug management programs for at-risk beneficiaries,* would require Part D prescription drug plans to provide drug management programs for Medicare beneficiaries who are at risk for prescription drug abuse. (Under current law, Part D plans are permitted but not required to establish such programs as of 2019). Based on an analysis of the number of plans currently providing those programs, CBO estimates that enacting H.R. 5675 would lower federal spending by $64 million over the 2019–2028 period by reducing the number of prescriptions filled and Medicare's payments for controlled substances.

*H.R. 5684, the Protecting Seniors from Opioid Abuse Act,* would expand medication therapy management programs under Medicare Part D to include beneficiaries who are at risk for prescription drug abuse. Because relatively few beneficiaries would be affected by this bill, CBO estimates that its enactment would not significantly affect direct spending for Part D.

*H.R. 5796, the Responsible Education Achieves Care and Healthy Outcomes for Users' Treatment Act of 2018,* would allow the Secretary of HHS to award grants to certain organizations that provide technical assistance and education to high-volume prescribers of opioids. The bill would appropriate $100 million for fiscal year 2019. Based on historical spending patterns for similar activities, CBO estimates that implementing H.R. 5796 would cost $100 million over the 2019–2028 period.

*H.R. 5798, the Opioid Screening and Chronic Pain Management Alternatives for Seniors Act,* would add an assessment of current opioid prescriptions and screening for opioid use disorder to the Welcome to Medicare Initial Preventive Physical Examination. Based on historical use of the examinations and pain management alternatives, CBO expects that enacting the bill would increase use of pain management services and estimates that direct spending would increase by $5 million over the 2019–2028 period.

*H.R. 5804, the Post-Surgical Injections as an Opioid Alternative Act,* would freeze the Medicare payment rate for certain analgesic injections provided in ambulatory surgical centers (ASCs). (For injections identified by specific billing codes, Medicare would pay the 2016 rate, which is higher than the current rate, during the 2020– 2024 period). Based on current utilization in the ASC setting, CBO estimates that enacting the legislation would increase direct spending by about $115 million over the

2019–2028 period. (If enacted, *H.R. 5804* also would affect spending subject to appropriation; see Table 3).

*H.R. 5809, the Postoperative Opioid Prevention Act of 2018,* would create an additional payment under Medicare for nonopioid analgesics. Under current law, certain new drugs and devices may receive an additional payment—separate from the bundled payment for a surgical procedure—in outpatient hospital departments and ambulatory surgical centers. The bill would allow nonopioid analgesics to qualify for a five-year period of additional payments. Based on its assessment of current spending for analgesics and on the probability of new nonopioid analgesics coming to market, CBO estimates that H.R. 5809 would increase direct spending by about $180 million over the 2019–2028 period.

Legislation Primarily Affecting the Food and Drug Administration. One bill related to the FDA would affect direct spending.

*H.R. 5333, the Over-the-Counter Monograph Safety, Innovation, and Reform Act of 2018,* would change the way that the FDA regulates the marketing of over-the-counter (OTC) medicines, and it would authorize that agency to grant 18 months of exclusive market protection for certain qualifying OTC drugs, thus delaying the entry of other versions of the same qualifying OTC product. Medicaid currently provides some coverage for OTC medicines, but only if a medicine is the least costly alternative in its drug class. On the basis of stakeholder feedback, CBO expects that delaying the availability of additional OTC versions of a drug would not significantly affect the average net price paid by Medicaid. As a result, CBO estimates that enacting H.R. 5333 would have a negligible effect on the federal budget. (If enacted, H.R. 5333 also would affect spending subject to appropriation; see Table 3).

Legislation with Revenue Effects. Two bills would affect revenues. However, CBO estimates that one bill, H.R. 5228, the Stop Counterfeit Drugs by Regulating and Enhancing Enforcement Now Act, would have only a negligible effect.

*5752, the Stop Illicit Drug Importation Act of 2018,* would amend the Federal, Food, Drug, and Cosmetic Act (FDCA) to strengthen the FDA's seizure powers and enhance its authority to detain, refuse, seize, or destroy illegal products offered for import. The legislation would subject more people to debarment under the FDCA and thus increase the potential for violations, and subsequently, the assessment of civil penalties, which are recorded in the budget as revenues. CBO estimates that those collections would result in an insignificant increase in revenues. Because H.R. 5752 would prohibit the importation of drugs that are in the process of being scheduled, it also could reduce amounts collected in customs duties. CBO anticipates that the result would be a negligible decrease in revenues. With those results taken together, CBO estimates, enacting H.R. 5752 would generate an insignificant net increase in revenues over the 2019–2028 period.

## Spending Subject to Appropriation

For this document, CBO has grouped bills with spending that would be subject to appropriation into four general categories:

- Bills that would have no budgetary effect,
- Bills with provisions that would authorize specified amounts to be appropriated (see Table 2),
- Bills with provisions for which CBO has estimated an au thorization of appropriations (see Table 3), and
- Bills with provisions that would affect spending subject to appropriation for which CBO has not yet completed an estimate.

No Budgetary Effect. CBO estimates that 6 of the 59 bills would have no effect on direct spending, revenues, or spending subject to appropriation.

*H.R. 3192, the CHIP Mental Health Parity Act,* would require all Children's Health Insurance Program (CHIP) plans to cover mental health and substance abuse treatment. In addition, states would not be allowed to impose financial or utilization limits on mental health treatment that are lower than limits placed on physical health treatment. Based on information from the Centers for Medicare and Medicaid Services, CBO estimates that enacting the bill would have no budgetary effect because all CHIP enrollees are already in plans that meet those requirements.

*H.R. 3331, a bill to amend title XI of the Social Security Act* to promote testing of incentive payments for behavioral health pro- viders for adoption and use of certified electronic health record technology, would give the Center for Medicare and Medicaid Innovation (CMMI) explicit authorization to test a program offering incentive payments to behavioral health providers that adopt and use certified electronic health record technology. Because it is already clear to CMMI that it has that authority, CBO estimates that enacting the legislation would not affect federal spending.

*H.R. 5202, the Ensuring Patient Access to Substance Use Disorder Treatments Act* of 2018, would clarify permission for pharmacists to deliver controlled substances to providers under certain circumstances. Because this provision would codify current practice, CBO estimates that H.R. 5202 would not affect direct spending or revenues during the 2019–2028 period.

*H.R. 5685, the Medicare Opioid Safety Education Act* of 2018, would require the Secretary of HHS to include information on opioid use, pain management, and nonopioid pain management treatments in future editions of Medicare & You, the program's handbook for beneficiaries, starting on January 1, 2019. Because H.R. 5685 would add information to an existing administrative document, CBO estimates that enacting the bill would have no budgetary effect.

*H.R. 5686, the Medicare Clear Health Options in Care for Enrollees Act* of 2018, would require prescription drug plans that provide coverage under Medicare Part D to furnish information to beneficiaries about the risks of opioid use and the availability of alternative treatments for pain. CBO estimates that enacting the bill would not affect direct spending because the required activities would not impose significant administrative costs.

**Table 2. Estimated spending subject to appropriation for bills with specified authorizations**

| | By fiscal year, in millions of dollars— | | | | | | |
|---|---|---|---|---|---|---|---|
| | 2018 | 2019 | 2020 | 2021 | 2022 | 2023 | 2019-2023 |
| Increases In Spending Subject To Appropriation | | | | | | | |
| H.R. 4684, Ensuring Access to Quality Sober Living Act: | | | | | | | |
| Authorization Level | 0 | 3 | 0 | 0 | 0 | 0 | 3 |
| Estimated Outlays | 0 | 1 | 2 | * | * | * | 3 |
| H.R. 5102, Substance Use Disorder Workforce Loan Repayment Act of 2018: | | | | | | | |
| Authorization Level | 0 | 25 | 25 | 25 | 25 | 25 | 125 |
| Estimated Outlays | 0 | 9 | 19 | 23 | 25 | 25 | 100 |
| H.R. 5176, Preventing Overdoses While in Emergency Rooms Act of 2018: | | | | | | | |
| Authorization Level | 0 | 50 | 0 | 0 | 0 | 0 | 50 |
| Estimated Outlays | 0 | 16 | 26 | 6 | 2 | 1 | 50 |
| H.R. 5197, Alternatives to Opioids (ALTO) in the Emergency Department Act: | | | | | | | |
| Authorization Level | 0 | 10 | 10 | 10 | 0 | 0 | 30 |
| Estimated Outlays | 0 | 3 | 8 | 10 | 7 | 2 | 30 |
| H.R. 5261, Treatment, Education, and Community Help to Combat Addiction Act of 2018: | | | | | | | |
| Authorization Level | 0 | 4 | 4 | 4 | 4 | 4 | 20 |
| Estimated Outlays | 0 | 1 | 3 | 4 | 4 | 4 | 16 |
| H.R. 5327, Comprehensive Opioid Recovery Centers Act of 2018: | | | | | | | |
| Authorization Level | 0 | 10 | 10 | 10 | 10 | 10 | 50 |
| Estimated Outlays | 0 | 3 | 8 | 10 | 10 | 10 | 41 |
| H.R. 5329, Poison Center Network Enhancement Act of 2018: Authorization Level | 0 | 30 | 30 | 30 | 30 | 30 | 151 |
| Estimated Outlays | 0 | 12 | 25 | 29 | 29 | 29 | 125 |
| H.R. 5353, Eliminating Opioid-Related Infectious Diseases Act of 2018: Authorization Level | 0 | 40 | 40 | 40 | 40 | 40 | 200 |
| Estimated Outlays | 0 | 15 | 34 | 38 | 39 | 40 | 166 |
| H.R. 5580, Surveillance and Testing of Opioids to Prevent Fentanyl Deaths Act of 2018: | | | | | | | |
| Authorization Level | 30 | 30 | 30 | 30 | 30 | 0 | 120 |
| Estimated Outlays | 0 | 11 | 25 | 29 | 29 | 19 | 113 |
| H.R. 5587, Peer Support Communities of Recovery Act: | | | | | | | |
| Authorization Level | 0 | 15 | 15 | 15 | 15 | 15 | 75 |
| Estimated Outlays | 0 | 5 | 13 | 14 | 15 | 15 | 62 |

Annual amounts may not sum to totals because of rounding. * = between zero and $500,000.

*H.R. 5716, the Commit to Opioid Medical Prescriber Accountability and Safety for Seniors Act,* would require the Secretary of HHS on an annual basis to identify high prescribers of opioids and furnish them with information about proper prescribing methods. Because HHS already has the capacity to meet those requirements, CBO estimates that enacting that provision would not impose additional administrative costs on the agency.

Specified Authorizations. Table 2 lists the ten bills that would authorize specified amounts to be appropriated over the 2019–2023 period. Spending from those authorized amounts would be subject to appropriation.

*H.R. 4684, the Ensuring Access to Quality Sober Living Act,* would direct the Secretary of HHS to develop and disseminate best practices for organizations that operate housing designed for people recovering from substance use disorders. The bill would authorize a total of $3 million over the 2019–2021 period for that purpose. Based on historical spending patterns for similar activities, CBO estimates that implementing H.R. 4684 would cost $3 million over the 2019–2023 period.

*H.R. 5102, the Substance Use Disorder Workforce Loan Repayment Act of 2018,* would establish a loan repayment program for mental health professionals who practice in areas with few mental health providers or with high rates of death from overdose and would authorize $25 million per year over the 2019–2028 period for that purpose. Based on historical spending patterns for similar activities, CBO estimates that implementing H.R. 5102 would cost $100 million over the 2019–2023 period; the remaining amounts would be spent in years after 2023.

*H.R. 5176, the Preventing Overdoses While in Emergency Rooms Act of 2018,* would require the Secretary of HHS to develop protocols and a grant program for health care providers to address the needs of people who survive a drug overdose, and it would authorize $50 million in 2019 for that purpose. Based on historical spending patterns for similar activities, CBO estimates that implementing H.R. 5176 would cost $50 million over the 2019–2023 period.

*H.R. 5197, the Alternatives to Opioids (ALTO) in the Emergency Department Act,* would direct the Secretary of HHS to carry out a demonstration program for hospitals and emergency departments to develop alternative protocols for pain management that limit the use of opioids and would authorize $10 million annually in grants for fiscal years

2019 through 2021. Based on historical spending patterns for similar programs, CBO estimates that implementing H.R. 5197 would cost $30 million over the 2019–2023 period.

**Table 3. Estimated spending subject to appropriation for bills with estimated authorizations**

| | By fiscal year, in millions of dollars— | | | | | | |
|---|---|---|---|---|---|---|---|
| | 2018 | 2019 | 2020 | 2021 | 2022 | 2023 | 2019-2023 |
| Increases In Spending Subject To Appropriation | | | | | | | |
| H.R. 449, Synthetic Drug Awareness Act of 2018 | | | | | | | |
| Estimated Authorization Level | 0 | * | * | * | 0 | 0 | 1 |
| Estimated Outlays | 0 | * | * | * | 0 | 0 | 1 |
| H.R. 4005, Medicaid Reentry Act: | | | | | | | |
| Estimated Authorization Level | * | * | 0 | 0 | 0 | 0 | * |
| Estimated Outlays | * | * | 0 | 0 | 0 | 0 | * |
| H.R. 4275, Empowering Pharmacists in the Fight Against Opioid Abuse Act: | | | | | | | |
| Estimated Authorization Level | 0 | * | * | * | * | * | * |
| Estimated Outlays | 0 | * | * | * | * | * | * |
| H.R. 5009, Jessie's Law: | | | | | | | |
| Estimated Authorization Level | 0 | * | * | * | * | * | * |
| Estimated Outlays | 0 | * | * | * | * | * | * |
| H.R. 5041, Safe Disposal of Unused Medication Act: | | | | | | | |
| Estimated Authorization Level | 0 | * | * | * | * | * | * |
| Estimated Outlays | 0 | * | * | * | * | * | * |
| H.R. 5272, Reinforcing Evidence-Based Standards Under Law in Treating Substance Abuse Act of 2018: | | | | | | | |
| Estimated Authorization Level | 0 | 1 | 1 | 1 | 1 | 1 | 4 |
| Estimated Outlays | 0 | 1 | 1 | 1 | 1 | 1 | 4 |
| H.R. 5333, Over-the-Counter Monograph Safety, Innovation, and Reform Act of 2018:[a] Food and Drug Administration: Collections from fees: | | | | | | | |
| Estimated Authorization Level | 0 | -22 | -22 | -26 | -35 | -42 | -147 |
| Estimated Outlays | 0 | -22 | -22 | -26 | -35 | -42 | -147 |
| Spending of fees: | | | | | | | |
| Estimated Authorization Level | 0 | 22 | 22 | 26 | 35 | 42 | 147 |
| Estimated Outlays | 0 | 6 | 17 | 30 | 44 | 41 | 137 |
| Net effect on FDA: | | | | | | | |
| Estimated Authorization Level | 0 | 0 | 0 | 0 | 0 | 0 | 0 |
| Estimated Outlays | 0 | -17 | -6 | 4 | 9 | * | -10 |

| | 2018 | 2019 | 2020 | 2021 | 2022 | 2023 | 2019-2023 |
|---|---|---|---|---|---|---|---|
| Government Accountability Office: | | | | | | | |
| Estimated Authorization Level | 0 | 0 | 0 | 0 | 0 | * | * |
| Estimated Outlays | 0 | 0 | 0 | 0 | 0 | * | * |
| **Total, H.R. 5333:** | | | | | | | |
| Estimated Authorization Level | 0 | 0 | 0 | 0 | 0 | * | * |
| Estimated Outlays | 0 | -17 | -6 | 4 | 9 | * | -10 |
| H.R. 5473, Better Pain Management Through Better Data Act of 2018: | | | | | | | |
| Estimated Authorization Level | 0 | * | * | * | * | * | * |
| Estimated Outlays | 0 | * | * | * | * | * | * |
| H.R. 5483, Special Registration for Telemedicine Clarification Act of 2018: | | | | | | | |
| Estimated Authorization Level | 0 | * | * | * | * | * | * |
| Estimated Outlays | 0 | * | * | * | * | * | * |
| H.R. 5554, Animal Drug and Animal Generic Drug User Fee Amendments of 2018: Collections from fees: | | | | | | | |
| Animal drug fees | 0 | -30 | -31 | -32 | -33 | -34 | -159 |
| Generic animal drug fees | 0 | -18 | -19 | -19 | -20 | -21 | -97 |
| Total, Estimated Authorization Level | 0 | -49 | -50 | -51 | -53 | -55 | -257 |
| Total, Estimated Outlays | 0 | -40 | -50 | -51 | -53 | -55 | -257 |
| Spending of fees: | | | | | | | |
| Animal drug fees | 0 | 30 | 31 | 32 | 33 | 34 | 159 |
| Generic animal drug fees | 0 | 18 | 19 | 19 | 20 | 21 | 97 |
| Total, Estimated Authorization Level | 0 | 49 | 50 | 51 | 53 | 55 | 257 |
| Total, Estimated Outlays | 0 | 39 | 47 | 51 | 52 | 54 | 243 |
| Net changes in fees: | | | | | | | |
| Estimated Authorization Level | 0 | 0 | 0 | 0 | 0 | 0 | 0 |
| Estimated Outlays | 0 | -10 | -3 | * | * | * | -14 |
| Other effects: | | | | | | | |
| Estimated Authorization Level | 0 | 3 | 1 | 1 | 1 | 1 | 6 |
| Estimated Outlays | 0 | 2 | 1 | 1 | 1 | 1 | 6 |
| **Total, H.R. 5554:** | | | | | | | |
| Estimated Authorization Level | 0 | 3 | 1 | 1 | 1 | 1 | 6 |
| Estimated Outlays | 0 | -8 | -2 | 1 | * | * | -8 |
| H.R. 5582, Abuse Deterrent Access Act of 2018: | | | | | | | |
| Estimated Authorization Level | 0 | 0 | * | 0 | 0 | 0 | * |
| Estimated Outlays | 0 | 0 | * | 0 | 0 | 0 | * |
| H.R. 5590, Opioid Addiction Action Plan Act: | | | | | | | |
| Estimated Authorization Level | * | * | * | * | * | * | * |
| Estimated Outlays | * | * | * | * | * | * | * |

**Table 3. (Continued)**

| | 2018 | 2019 | 2020 | 2021 | 2022 | 2023 | 2019-2023 |
|---|---|---|---|---|---|---|---|
| H.R. 5687, Securing Opioids and Unused Narcotics with Deliberate Disposal and Packaging Act of 2018: | | | | | | | |
| Estimated Authorization Level | 0 | * | * | * | * | * | * |
| Estimated Outlays | 0 | * | * | * | * | * | * |
| H.R. 5715, Strengthening Partnerships to Prevent Opioid Abuse Act: | | | | | | | |
| Estimated Authorization Level | 0 | 2 | 2 | 2 | 2 | 2 | 9 |
| Estimated Outlays | 0 | 2 | 2 | 2 | 2 | 2 | 9 |
| H.R. 5789, a bill to require the Secretary of Health and Human Services to issue guidance to improve care for infants with neonatal abstinence syndrome and their mothers, and to require the Comptroller General of the United States to conduct a study on gaps in Medicaid coverage for pregnant and postpartum women with substance use disorder: | | | | | | | |
| Estimated Authorization Level | 0 | 2 | 0 | 0 | 0 | 0 | 2 |
| Estimated Outlays | 0 | 2 | 0 | 0 | 0 | 0 | 2 |
| H.R. 5795, Overdose Prevention and Patient Safety Act: | | | | | | | |
| Estimated Authorization Level | 0 | 1 | 0 | 0 | 0 | 0 | 1 |
| Estimated Outlays | 0 | 1 | 0 | 0 | 0 | 0 | 1 |
| H.R. 5800, Medicaid IMD ADDITIONAL INFO Act: | | | | | | | |
| Estimated Authorization Level | 0 | 1 | 0 | 0 | 0 | 0 | 1 |
| Estimated Outlays | 0 | * | * | 0 | 0 | 0 | 1 |
| H.R. 5804, Post-Surgical Injections as an Opioid Alternative Act:[a] | | | | | | | |
| Estimated Authorization Level | 0 | 0 | 0 | 0 | 1 | 1 | 1 |
| Estimated Outlays | 0 | 0 | 0 | 0 | 1 | 1 | 1 |
| H.R. 5811, a bill to amend the Federal Food, Drug, and Cosmetic Act with respect to postapproval study requirements for certain controlled substances, and for other purposes: | | | | | | | |
| Estimated Authorization Level | 0 | * | * | * | * | * | * |
| Estimated Outlays | 0 | * | * | * | * | * | * |

Annual amounts may not sum to totals because of rounding. * = between ¥$500,000 and $500,000.
[a] This bill also would affect mandatory spending (see Table 1).

*H.R. 5261, the Treatment, Education, and Community Help to Combat Addiction Act of 2018,* would direct the Secretary of HHS to designate regional centers of excellence to improve the training of health professionals who treat substance use disorders. The bill would authorize $4 million annually for grants to those programs over the 2019–2023 period. Based on historical spending patterns for similar activities, CBO estimates that implementing H.R. 5261 would cost $16 million over the

2019–2023 period; the remaining amounts would be spent in years after 2023.

*H.R. 5327, the Comprehensive Opioid Recovery Centers Act of 2018,* would direct the Secretary of HHS to award grants to at least 10 providers that offer treatment services for people with opioid use disorder, and it would authorize $10 million per year over the 2019–2023 period for that purpose. Based on historical spending patterns for similar activities, CBO estimates that implementing H.R. 5327 would cost $41 million over the 2019–2023 period; the remaining amounts would be spent in years after 2023.

*H.R. 5329, the Poison Center Network Enhancement Act of 2018,* would reauthorize the poison control center toll-free number, national media campaign, and grant program under the Public Health Service Act. Among other actions, H.R. 5329 would increase the share of poison control center funding that could be provided by federal grants. The bill would authorize a total of about $30 million per year over the 2019–2023 period. Based on historical spending patterns for similar activities, CBO estimates that implementing H.R. 5329 would cost $125 million over the 2019–2023 period; the remaining amounts would be spent in years after 2023.

*H.R 5353, the Eliminating Opioid Related Infectious Diseases Act of 2018,* would amend Public Health Service Act by broadening the focus of surveillance and education programs from preventing and treating hepatitis C virus to preventing and treating infections associated with injection drug use. It would authorize $40 million per year over 2019–2023 period for that purpose. Based on historical spending patterns for similar activities, CBO estimates that implementing H.R. 5353 would cost $166 million over the 2019–2023 period; the remaining amounts would be spent in years after 2023.

*H.R. 5580, the Surveillance and Testing of Opioids to Prevent Fentanyl Deaths Act of 2018,* would establish a grant program for public health laboratories that conduct testing for fentanyl and other synthetic opioids. It also would direct the Centers for Disease Control and Prevention to expand its drug surveillance program, with a particular focus on collecting data on fentanyl. The bill would authorize a total of $30 million per year over the 2018–2022 period for those activities. Based on historical spending patterns for similar activities, CBO estimates that implementing H.R. 5580 would cost $113 million over the 2019–2023 period; the remaining amounts would be spent in years after 2023.

*H.R. 5587, Peer Support Communities of Recovery Act,* would direct the Secretary of HHS to award grants to nonprofit organizations that support community-based, peer-delivered support, including technical support for the establishment of recovery community organizations, independent, nonprofit groups led by people in recovery and their families. The bill would authorize $15 million per year for the 2019–2023 period. Based on historical spending patterns for similar activities, CBO estimates that implementing

H.R. 5587 would cost $62 million over the 2019–2023 period; the remaining amounts would be spent in years after 2023.

Estimated Authorizations. Table 3 shows CBO's estimates of the appropriations that would be necessary to implement 19 of the bills. Spending would be subject to appropriation of those amounts.

*H.R. 449, the Synthetic Drug Awareness Act of 2018,* would require the Surgeon General to report to the Congress on the health effects of synthetic psychoactive drugs on children between the ages of 12 and 18. Based on spending patterns for similar activities, CBO estimates that implementing H.R. 449 would cost approximately $1 million over the 2019–2023 period.

*H.R. 4005, the Medicaid Reentry Act,* would direct the Secretary of HHS to convene a group of stakeholders to develop and report to the Congress on best practices for addressing issues related to health care faced by those returning from incarceration to their communities. The bill also would require the Secretary to issue a letter to state Medicaid directors about relevant demonstration projects. Based on an analysis of anticipated workload, CBO estimates that implementing H.R. 4005 would cost less than $500,000 over the 2018–2023 period.

*H.R. 4275, the Empowering Pharmacists in the Fight Against Opioid Abuse Act,* would require the Secretary of HHS to develop and disseminate materials for training pharmacists, health care practitioners, and the public about the circumstances under which a pharmacist may decline to fill a prescription. Based on historical spending patterns for similar activities, CBO estimates that costs to the federal government for the development and distribution of those materials would not be significant.

*H.R. 5009, Jessie's Law,* would require HHS, in collaboration with outside experts, to develop best practices for displaying information about opioid use disorder in a patient's medical record. HHS also would be required to develop and disseminate written materials annually to health care providers about what disclosures could be made while still complying with federal laws that govern health care privacy. Based on spending patterns for similar activities, CBO estimates that implementing H.R. 5009 would have an insignificant effect on spending over the 2019–2023 period.

*H.R. 5041, the Safe Disposal of Unused Medication Act,* would re quire hospice programs to have written policies and procedures for the disposal of controlled substances after a patient's death. Certain licensed employees of hospice programs would be permitted to assist in the disposal of controlled substances that were lawfully dispensed. Using information from the Department of Justice (DOJ), CBO estimates that implementing the bill would cost less than $500,000 over the 2019–2023 period.

*H.R. 5272, the Reinforcing Evidence-Based Standards Under Law in Treating Substance Abuse Act of 2018,* would require the newly established National Mental Health and Substance Use Policy Laboratory to issue guidance to applicants for SAMHSA grants that support evidence-based practices. Using information from HHS about the historical cost of similar activities, CBO estimates that enacting this bill would cost approximately $4 million over the 2019–2023 period.

*H.R. 5333, the Over-the-Counter Monograph Safety, Innovation, and Reform Act of 2018,* would change the FDA's oversight of the commercial marketing of OTC medicines and authorize the collection and spending of fees through 2023 to cover the costs of expediting the FDA's administrative procedures for certain regulatory activities relating to OTC products. Under H.R. 5333, CBO estimates, the FDA would assess about $147 million in fees over the 2019–2023 period that could be collected and made available for obligation only to the extent and in the amounts provided in advance in appropriation acts. Because the FDA could spend those fees, CBO estimates that the estimated budget authority for collections and spending would offset each other exactly in each year, although CBO expects that spending initially would lag behind collections. Assuming appropriation action consistent with the bill, CBO estimates that implementing H.R. 5333 would reduce net discretionary outlays by $10 million over the 2019–2023 period, primarily because of that lag. The bill also would require the Government Accountability Office to study exclusive market protections for certain qualifying OTC drugs authorized by the bill—a provision that CBO estimates would cost less than $500,000. (If enacted,

H.R. 5333 also would affect mandatory spending; see Table 1).

*H.R. 5473, the Better Pain Management through Better Data Act of 2018,* would require that the FDA conduct a public meeting and issue guidance to industry addressing data collection and labeling for medical products that reduce pain while enabling the reduction, replacement, or avoidance of oral opioids. Using information from the agency, CBO estimates that implementing H.R. 5473 would cost about $1 million over the 2019–2023 period.

*H.R. 5483, the Special Registration for Telemedicine Clarification Act of 2018,* would direct DOJ, within one year of the bill's enactment, to issue regulations concerning the practice of telemedicine (for remote diagnosis and treatment of patients). Using information from DOJ, CBO estimates that implementing the bill would cost less than $500,000 over the 2019–2023 period.

*H.R. 5554, the Animal Drug and Animal Generic Drug User Fee Amendments of 2018,* would authorize the FDA to collect and spend fees to cover the cost of expedited approval for the development and marketing of certain drugs for use in animals. The legislation would extend through fiscal year 2023, and make several changes to, the FDA's existing approval processes and fee programs for brand-name and generic veterinary drugs, which expire at the end of fiscal year 2018. CBO estimates that implementing H.R. 5554 would reduce net discretionary outlays by $8 million over the 2019–2023 period, primarily because the spending of fees lags somewhat behind their collection.

Fees authorized under the bill would supplement funds appropriated to cover the FDA's cost of reviewing certain applications and investigational submissions for brand-name and generic drugs for use in animals. Those fees could be collected and made available for obligation only to the extent and in the amounts provided in advance in appropriation acts. Under H.R. 5554, CBO estimates, the FDA would assess about $257 million in fees over the 2019– 2023 period. Because the FDA could spend those funds, CBO estimates that budget authority for collections and spending would offset each other exactly in each year. CBO estimates that the delay between collecting and spending fees under the reauthorized programs would reduce net discretionary outlays by $14 million over the 2019–2023 period, assuming appropriation actions consistent with the bill.

Enacting H.R. 5554 would increase the FDA's workload because the legislation would expand eligibility for conditional approval for certain drugs. The agency's administrative costs also would increase because of regulatory activities required by a provision concerning petitions for additives intended for use in animal food. H.R. 5554 also would require the FDA to publish guidance or produce regulations on a range of topics, transmit a report to the Congress, and hold public meetings. CBO expects that the costs associated with those activities would not be covered by fees, and it estimates that implementing such provisions would cost $6 million over the 2019–2023 period.

*H.R. 5582, the Abuse Deterrent Access Act of 2018,* would require the Secretary of HHS to report to the Congress on existing barriers to access to "abuse-deterrent opioid formulations" by Medicare Part C and D beneficiaries. Such formulations make the drugs more difficult to dissolve for injection, for example, and thus can impede their abuse. Assuming the availability of appropriated funds and based on historical spending patterns for similar activities, CBO estimates that implementing the legislation would cost less than $500,000 over the 2019–2023 period.

*H.R. 5590, the Opioid Addiction Action Plan Act,* would require the Secretary of HHS to develop an action plan by January 1, 2019, for increasing access to medication-assisted treatment among Medicare and Medicaid enrollees. The bill also would require HHS to convene a stakeholder meeting and issue a request for information within three months of enactment, and to submit a report to the Congress by June 1, 2019. Based on historical spending patterns for similar activities, CBO estimates that implementing H.R. 5590 would cost approximately $2 million over the 2019–2023 period.

*H.R. 5687, the Securing Opioids and Unused Narcotics with De liberate Disposal and Packaging Act of 2018,* would permit the FDA to require certain packaging and disposal technologies, controls, or measures to mitigate the risk of abuse and misuse of drugs. Based on information from the FDA, CBO estimates that implementing H.R. 5687 would not significantly affect spending over the 2019–2023 period. This bill would also require that the GAO study the effectiveness and use of packaging technologies for controlled substances—a provision that CBO estimates would cost less than $500,000.

*H.R. 5715, the Strengthening Partnerships to Prevent Opioid Abuse Act,* would require the Secretary of HHS to establish a secure Internet portal to allow HHS, Medicare Advantage plans, and Medicare Part D plans to exchange information about fraud, waste, and abuse among providers and suppliers no later than two years after enactment. H.R. 5715 also would require organizations with Medicare Advantage contracts to submit information on investigations related to providers suspected of prescribing large volumes of opioids through a process established by the Secretary no later than January 2021. Based on historical spending patterns for similar activities, CBO estimates that implementing H.R. 5715 would cost approximately $9 million over the 2019–2023 period.

*H.R. 5789, a bill to require the Secretary of Health and Human Services to issue guidance to improve care for infants with neonatal abstinence syndrome and their mothers, and to require the Comptroller General of the United States to conduct a study on gaps in Medicaid coverage for pregnant and postpartum women with substance use disorder,* would direct the Secretary of HHS to issue guidance to states on best practices under Medicaid and CHIP for treating infants with neonatal abstinence syndrome. H.R. 5789 also would direct the Government Accountability Office to study Medicaid coverage for pregnant and postpartum women with substance use disorders. Based on information from HHS and historical spending patterns for similar activities, CBO estimates that enacting H.R. 5789 would cost approximately $2 million over the 2019– 2023 period.

*H.R. 5795, the Overdose Prevention and Patient Safety Act,* would amend the Public Health Service Act so that requirements pertaining to the confidentiality and disclosure of medical records relating to substance use disorders align with the provisions of the Health Insurance Portability and Accountability Act of 1996. The bill would require the Office of the Secretary of HHS to issue regulations prohibiting discrimination based on data disclosed from such medical records, to issue regulations requiring covered entities to provide written notice of privacy practices, and to develop model training programs and materials for health care providers and patients and their families. Based on spending patterns for similar activities, CBO estimates that implementing H.R. 5795 would cost approximately $1 million over the 2019–2023 period.

*H.R. 5800, Medicaid IMD ADDITIONAL INFO Act,* would direct the Medicaid and CHIP Payment and Access Commission to study institutions for mental diseases in a representative sample of states. Based on information from the commission about the cost of similar work, CBO estimates that implementing H.R. 5800 would cost about $1 million over the 2019–2023 period.

*H.R. 5804, the Post-Surgical Injections as an Opioid Alternative Act,* would freeze the Medicare payment rate for certain analgesic injections provided in ambulatory surgical centers. The bill also would mandate two studies of Medicare coding and payments arising from enactment of this legislation. Based on the cost of similar activities, CBO estimates that those reports would cost $1 million over the 2019–2023 period (If enacted, H.R. 5804 also would affect mandatory spending; see Table 1).

*5811, a bill to amend the Federal Food, Drug, and Cosmetic Act with respect to postapproval study requirements for certain controlled substances, and for other purposes,* would allow the FDA to require that pharmaceutical manufacturers study certain drugs after they are approved to assess any potential reduction in those drugs' effectiveness for the conditions of use prescribed, recommended, or suggested in labeling. CBO anticipates that implementing H.R. 5811 would not significantly affect the FDA's costs over the 2019–2023 period.

Other Authorizations. The following nine bills would increase au thorization levels, but CBO has not completed estimates of amounts. All authorizations would be subject to future appropriation action.

- H.R. 4284, Indexing Narcotics, Fentanyl, and Opioids Act of 2017
- H.R. 5002, Advancing Cutting Edge Research Act
- H.R. 5228, Stop Counterfeit Drugs by Regulating and Enhancing Enforcement Now Act (see Table 1 for an estimate of the revenue effects of H.R. 5228)
- H.R. 5752, Stop Illicit Drug Importation Act of 2018 (see Table 1 for an estimate of the revenue effects of H.R. 5752)
- H.R. 5799, Medicaid DRUG Improvement Act (see Table 1 for an estimate of the direct spending effects of H.R. 5799)
- H.R. 5801, Medicaid Providers and Pharmacists Are Required to Note Experiences in Record Systems to Help In-Need Patients (PARTNERSHIP) Act (see Table 1 for an estimate of the direct spending effects of H.R. 5801)
- H.R. 5806, 21st Century Tools for Pain and Addiction Treatments Act
- H.R. 5808, Medicaid Pharmaceutical Home Act of 2018 (see Table 1 for an estimate of the direct spending effects of H.R. 5808)
- H.R. 5812, Creating Opportunities that Necessitate New and Enhanced Connections That Improve Opioid Navigation Strategies Act (CONNECTIONS) Act

Pay-As-You-Go considerations: The Statutory Pay-As-You-Go Act of 2010 establishes budget-reporting and enforcement procedures for legislation affecting direct spending or revenues. Twenty-two of the bills discussed in this document contain direct spending or revenues and are subject to pay-as-you-go procedures.

Details about the amount of direct spending and revenues in those bills can be found in Table 1.

Increase in long-term direct spending and deficits: CBO estimates that enacting H.R. 4998, the Health Insurance for Former Foster Youth Act, would increase net direct spending by more than $2.5 billion and on-budget deficits by more than $5 billion in at least one of the four consecutive 10-year periods beginning in 2029. CBO estimates that none of the remaining 58 bills included in this estimate would increase net direct spending by more than $2.5 billion or on-budget deficits by more than $5 billion in any of the four consecutive 10-year periods beginning in 2029.

Mandates: One of the 59 bills included in this document, H.R. 5795, would impose both intergovernmental and private-sector mandates as defined in UMRA. CBO estimates that the costs of that bill's mandates on public and private entities would fall below UMRA's thresholds ($80 million and $160 million, respectively, for publicand private-sector entities in 2018, adjusted annually for inflation).

In addition, five bills would impose private-sector mandates as defined in UMRA. CBO estimates that the costs of the mandates in three of those bills (H.R. 5333, H.R. 5554, and H.R. 5811) would fall below the UMRA threshold. Because CBO does not know how federal agencies would implement new authority granted in the other two of those five bills, H.R. 5228 and 5687, CBO cannot determine whether the costs of their mandates would exceed the threshold.

For large entitlement grant programs, including Medicaid and CHIP, UMRA defines an increase in the stringency of conditions on states or localities as an intergovernmental mandate if the affected governments lack authority to offset those costs while continuing to provide required services. Because states possess significant flexibility to alter their responsibilities within Medicaid and CHIP, the requirements imposed by various bills in the markup on state administration of those programs would not constitute mandates as defined in UMRA.

## Mandates Affecting Public and Private Entities

*H.R. 5795, the Overdose Prevention and Patient Safety Act,* would impose intergovernmental and private-sector mandates by requiring entities that provide treatment for substance use disorders to notify patients of their privacy rights and also to notify patients in the event that the confidentiality of their records is breached. In certain circumstances, H.R. 5795 also would prohibit public and private entities from denying entry to treatment on the basis of information in patient health records. Those requirements would either supplant or narrowly expand responsibilities under existing law, and compliance with them would not impose significant additional costs. CBO estimates that the costs of the mandates would fall below the annual thresholds established in UMRA.

## Mandates Affecting Private Entities

Five bills included in this document would impose private-sector mandates:

*H.R. 5228, the Stop Counterfeit Drugs by Regulating and Enhancing Enforcement Now Act,* would require drug distributors to cease distributing any drug that the Secretary of HHS determines might present an imminent or substantial hazard to public health. CBO cannot determine what drugs could be subject to such an order nor can it determine how private entities would respond. Consequently, CBO cannot determine whether the aggregate cost of the mandate would exceed the annual threshold for private-sector mandates.

*H.R. 5333, the Over-the-Counter Monograph Safety, Innovation, and Reform Act of 2018,* would require developers and manufacturers of OTC drugs to pay certain fees to the FDA. CBO estimates that about $30 million would be collected each year, on average, for a total of $147 million over the 2019–2023 period. Those amounts would not exceed the annual threshold for private-sector mandates in any year during that period.

*H.R. 5554, the Animal Drug and Animal Generic Drug User Fee Amendments of 2018,* would require developers and manufacturers of brand-name and generic veterinary drugs to pay application, product, establishment, and sponsor fees to the FDA. CBO estimates that about $51 million would be collected annually, on average, for a total of $257 million over the 2019–2023 period. Those amounts would not exceed the annual threshold for private-sector mandates in any year during that period.

*H.R. 5687, the Securing Opioids and Unused Narcotics with De liberate Disposal and Packaging Act of 2018,* would permit the Secretary of HHS to require drug developers and manufacturers to implement new packaging and disposal technology for certain drugs. Based on information from the agency, CBO expects that the Secretary would use the new regulatory authority provided in the bill; however, it is uncertain how or when those requirements would be implemented. Consequently, CBO cannot determine whether the aggregate cost of the mandate would exceed the annual threshold for private entities.

*5811, a bill to amend the Federal Food, Drug, and Cosmetic Act with respect to postapproval study requirements for certain controlled substances, and for other purposes,* would expand an existing mandate that requires drug developers to conduct postapproval studies or clinical trials for certain drugs. Under current law, in certain instances, the FDA can require studies or clinical trials after a drug has been approved. H.R. 5811 would permit the FDA to use that authority if the reduction in a drug's effectiveness meant that its benefits no longer outweighed its costs. CBO estimates that the incremental cost of the mandate would fall below the annual threshold established in UMRA because of the small number of drugs affected and the narrow expansion of the authority that exists under current law.

None of the remaining 53 bills included in this document would impose an intergovernmental or private-sector mandate.

Previous CBO estimate: On June 6, 2018, CBO issued an estimate for seven opioid-related bills ordered reported by the House Committee on Ways and Means on May 16, 2018. Two of those bills contain provisions that are identical or similar to the legislation ordered reported by the

Committee on Energy and Commerce, and for those provisions, CBO's estimates are the same.

In particular, five bills listed in this estimate contain provisions that are identical or similar to those in several sections of H.R. 5773, the Preventing Addiction for Susceptible Seniors Act of 2018:

- H.R. 5675, which would require prescription drug plans to implement drug management programs, is identical to section 2 of H.R. 5773.
- H.R. 4841, regarding electronic prior authorization for prescriptions under Medicare's Part D, is similar to section 3 of H.R. 5773.
- H.R. 5715, which would mandate the creation of a new Inter- net portal to allow various stakeholders to exchange information, is identical to section 4 of H.R. 5773.
- H.R. 5684, which would expand medication therapy management, is the same as section 5 of H.R. 5773.
- H.R. 5716, regarding prescriber notification, is identical to section 6 of H.R. 5773.

In addition, in this estimate, a provision related to Medicare ben eficiary education in H.R. 5686, the Medicare Clear Health Options in Care for Enrollees Act of 2018, is the same as a provision in section 2 of H.R. 5775, the Providing Reliable Options for Patients and Educational Resources Act of 2018, in CBO's estimate for the Committee on Ways and Means.

Estimate prepared by: Federal Costs: Rebecca Yip (Centers for Disease Control and Prevention), Mark Grabowicz (Drug Enforcement Agency), Julia Christensen, Ellen Werble (Food and Drug Administration), Emily King, Andrea Noda, Lisa Ramirez-Branum, Robert Stewart (Medicaid and Children's Health Insurance Program), Philippa Haven, Lara Robillard, Colin Yee, Rebecca Yip (Medicare), Philippa Haven (National Institutes of Health), Alice Burns, Andrea Noda (Office of the Secretary of the Department of Health and Human Services), Philippa Haven, Lori

Housman, Emily King (Substance Abuse and Mental Health Services Administration, Health Resources and Services Administration); Federal Revenues: Jacob Fabian, Peter Huether, and Cecilia Pastrone; Fact Checking: Zachary Byrum and Kate Kelly; Mandates: Andrew Laughlin.

Estimate reviewed by: Tom Bradley, Chief Health Systems and Medicare Cost Estimates Unit; Chad M. Chirico, Chief, Low-Income Health Programs and Prescription Drugs Cost Estimates Unit; Sarah Masi, Special Assistant for Health; Susan Willie, Chief, Mandates Unit; Leo Lex, Deputy Assistant Director for Budget Analysis; Theresa A. Gullo, Assistant Director for Budget Analysis.

## FEDERAL MANDATES STATEMENT

The Committee adopts as its own the estimate of Federal mandates prepared by the Director of the Congressional Budget Office pursuant to section 423 of the Unfunded Mandates Reform Act.

## STATEMENT OF GENERAL PERFORMANCE GOALS AND OBJECTIVES

Pursuant to clause 3(c)(4) of rule XIII, the general performance goal or objective of this legislation is to help facilitate communication among MA organizations, Part D plan sponsors, and CMS relating to substantiated fraud, waste, and abuse investigations.

## DUPLICATION OF FEDERAL PROGRAMS

Pursuant to clause 3(c)(5) of rule XIII, no provision H.R. 5715 is known to be duplicative of another Federal program, including any program that was included in a report to Congress pursuant to section 21 of

Public Law 111–139 or the most recent Catalog of Federal Domestic Assistance.

## COMMITTEE COST ESTIMATE

Pursuant to clause 3(d)(1) of rule XIII, the Committee adopts as its own the cost estimate prepared by the Director of the Congressional Budget Office pursuant to section 402 of the Congressional Budget Act of 1974.

## EARMARK, LIMITED TAX BENEFITS, AND LIMITED TARIFF BENEFITS

Pursuant to clause 9(e), 9(f), and 9(g) of rule XXI, the Committee finds that H.R. 5715 contains no earmarks, limited tax benefits, or limited tariff benefits.

## DISCLOSURE OF DIRECTED RULE MAKINGS

Pursuant to section 3(i) of H. Res. 5, the following directed rule makings are contained in H.R. 5715:

- Section 2(a)(i)(1)(C): The Secretary shall, through rule making, specify what constitutes substantiated fraud, waste, and abuse, using guidance such as what is provided in the Medicare Program Integrity Manual 4.7.1.
- Section 2(b)(5)(C): The Secretary shall, pursuant to rulemaking, (i) specify a definition for the term "high volume of opioids" and a method for determining if a provider of services prescribes such a high volume; and (ii) establish the process described in

subparagraph (B) and the types of information that shall be submitted through such process.

## ADVISORY COMMITTEE STATEMENT

No advisory committees within the meaning of section 5(b) of the Federal Advisory Committee Act were created by this legislation.

## APPLICABILITY TO LEGISLATIVE BRANCH

The Committee finds that the legislation does not relate to the terms and conditions of employment or access to public services or accommodations within the meaning of section 102(b)(3) of the Con gressional Accountability Act.

## SECTION-BY-SECTION ANALYSIS OF THE LEGISLATION

### Section 1. Short Title

Section 1 provides that the Act may be cited as the "Strengthening Partnerships to Prevent Opioid Abuse Act."

### Section 2. Program Integrity Transparency Measures under Medicare Parts C and D

Section 2 directs the Secretary to establish a secure online portal to improve communication between CMS, MA plans, Part D plans, and the Medicare Drug Integrity Contractor (MEDIC) no later than two years after enactment. The Secretary is also required to submit quarterly reports to plans including pertinent information such as trends in identifying suspicious activity and information on fraud, waste, and abuse schemes. By no later than January 1, 2021, the Secretary shall also establish a process for plans to submit information on investigations and other actions relating to high volumes of opioid prescriptions.

## Changes in Existing Law Made by the Bill, as Reported

In compliance with clause 3(e) of rule XIII of the Rules of the House of Representatives, changes in existing law made by the bill, as reported, are shown as follows (new matter is printed in italic and existing law in which no change is proposed is shown in roman): Social Security Act Title XVIII—Health Insurance For The Aged And

Disabled Part C—Medicare+Choice Program Contracts With Medicare+Choice Organizations

## Sec. 1857. (a) In General

The Secretary shall not permit the election under section 1851 of a Medicare+Choice plan offered by a Medicare+Choice organization under this part, and no payment shall be made under section 1853 to an organization, unless the Secretary has entered into a contract under this section with the organization with respect to the offering of such plan. Such a contract with an organization may cover more than 1 Medicare+Choice plan. Such contract shall provide that the organization agrees to comply with the applicable requirements and standards of this part and the terms and conditions of payment as provided for in this part.

(b) MINIMUM ENROLLMENT REQUIREMENTS.—

(1) IN GENERAL.—Subject to paragraph (2), the Secretary may not enter into a contract under this section with a Medicare+Choice organization unless the organization has—

(A) at least 5,000 individuals (or 1,500 individuals in the case of an organization that is a provider-sponsored organization) who are receiving health benefits through the organization, or

(B) at least 1,500 individuals (or 500 individuals in the case of an organization that is a provider-sponsored organization) who are receiving health benefits through the organization if the organization primarily serves individuals residing outside of urbanized areas.

(2) APPLICATION TO MSA PLANS.—In applying paragraph (1) in the case of a Medicare+Choice organization that is offering an MSA plan, paragraph (1) shall be applied by substituting covered lives for individuals.

(3) ALLOWING TRANSITION.—The Secretary may waive the requirement of paragraph (1) during the first 3 contract years with respect to an organization.

(c) CONTRACT PERIOD AND EFFECTIVENESS.—

(1) PERIOD.—Each contract under this section shall be for a term of at least 1 year, as determined by the Secretary, and may be made automatically renewable from term to term in the absence of notice by either party of intention to terminate at the end of the current term.

(2) TERMINATION AUTHORITY.—In accordance with procedures established under subsection (h), the Secretary may at any time terminate any such contract if the Secretary determines that the organization—

(A) has failed substantially to carry out the contract;

(B) is carrying out the contract in a manner inconsistent with the efficient and effective administration of this part; or

(C) no longer substantially meets the applicable conditions of this part.

(3) EFFECTIVE DATE OF CONTRACTS.—The effective date of any contract executed pursuant to this section shall be specified in the contract, except that in no case shall a contract under this section which provides for coverage under an MSA plan be effective before January 1999 with respect to such coverage.

(4) PREVIOUS TERMINATIONS.—

(A) IN GENERAL.—The Secretary may not enter into a contract with a Medicare+Choice organization if a previous contract with that organization under this section was terminated at the request of the organization within the preceding 2-year period, except as provided in subparagraph (B) and except in such other circumstances which warrant special consideration, as determined by the Secretary.

(B) EARLIER RE-ENTRY PERMITTED WHERE CHANGE IN PAYMENT POLICY.—Subparagraph (A) shall not apply with respect to the offering by a Medicare+Choice organization of a Medicare+Choice plan in a Medicare+Choice payment area if during the 6-month period beginning on the date the organization notified the Secretary of the intention to terminate the most recent previous contract, there was a legislative change enacted (or a regulatory change adopted) that has the effect of increasing payment amounts under section 1853 for that Medicare+Choice payment area.

(5) CONTRACTING AUTHORITY.—The authority vested in the Secretary by this part may be performed without regard to such provisions of law or regulations relating to the making, performance, amendment, or modification of contracts of the United States as the Secretary may determine to be inconsistent with the furtherance of the purpose of this title.

(d) PROTECTIONS AGAINST FRAUD AND BENEFICIARY PROTECTIONS.—

(1) PERIODIC AUDITING.—The Secretary shall provide for the annual auditing of the financial records (including data relating to medicare utilization and costs, including allowable costs under section 1858(c)) of at least one-third of the Medicare+Choice organizations offering Medicare+Choice plans under this part. The Comptroller General shall monitor auditing activities conducted under this subsection.

(2) INSPECTION AND AUDIT.—Each contract under this section shall provide that the Secretary, or any person or organization designated by the Secretary—

(A) shall have the right to timely inspect or otherwise evaluate (i) the quality, appropriateness, and timeliness of services performed under the contract, and (ii) the facilities of the organization when there is reasonable evidence of some need for such inspection, and

(B) shall have the right to timely audit and inspect any books and records of the Medicare+Choice organization that pertain (i) to the ability of the organization to bear the risk of potential financial losses, or (ii) to services performed or determinations of amounts payable under the contract.

(3) ENROLLEE NOTICE AT TIME OF TERMINATION.—Each contract under this section shall require the organization to provide (and pay for) written notice in advance of the contract's termination, as well as a description of alternatives for obtaining benefits under this title, to each individual enrolled with the organization under this part.

(4) DISCLOSURE.—

(A) IN GENERAL.—Each Medicare+Choice organization shall, in accordance with regulations of the Secretary, report to the Secretary financial information which shall include the following:

(i) Such information as the Secretary may require demonstrating that the organization has a fiscally sound operation.

(ii) A copy of the report, if any, filed with the Secretary containing the information required to be reported under section 1124 by disclosing entities.

(iii) A description of transactions, as specified by the Secretary, between the organization and a party in interest. Such transactions shall include—

(I) any sale or exchange, or leasing of any property between the organization and a party in interest;

(II) any furnishing for consideration of goods, services (including management services), or facilities between the organization and a party in interest, but not including salaries paid to employees for services provided in the normal course of their employment and health services provided to members by hospitals and other providers and by staff, medical group (or groups), individual practice association (or associations), or any combination thereof; and

(III) any lending of money or other extension of credit between an organization and a party in interest.

The Secretary may require that information reported respecting an organization which controls, is controlled by, or is under common control with, another entity be in the form of a consolidated financial statement for the organization and such entity.

(B) PARTY IN INTEREST DEFINED.—For the purposes of this paragraph, the term "party in interest" means—

(i) any director, officer, partner, or employee responsible for management or administration of a Medicare+Choice organization, any person who is directly or indirectly the beneficial owner of more than 5 percent of the equity of the organization, any person who is the beneficial owner of a mortgage, deed of trust, note, or other interest secured by, and valuing more than 5 percent of the organization, and, in the case of a Medicare+Choice organization organized as a nonprofit corporation, an incorporator or member of such corporation under applicable State corporation law;

(ii) any entity in which a person described in clause (i)—

(I) is an officer or director;

(II) is a partner (if such entity is organized as a partnership);

(III) has directly or indirectly a beneficial interest of more than 5 percent of the equity; or

(IV) has a mortgage, deed of trust, note, or other interest valuing more than 5 percent of the assets of such entity;

(iii) any person directly or indirectly controlling, controlled by, or under common control with an organization; and

(iv) any spouse, child, or parent of an individual described in clause (i).

(C) ACCESS TO INFORMATION.—Each Medicare+Choice organization shall make the information reported pursuant to subparagraph (A) available to its enrollees upon reasonable request.

(5) LOAN INFORMATION.—The contract shall require the organization to notify the Secretary of loans and other special financial arrangements which are made between the organization and subcontractors, affiliates, and related parties.

(6) REVIEW TO ENSURE COMPLIANCE WITH CARE MANAGEMENT REQUIREMENTS FOR SPECIALIZED MEDICARE ADVANTAGE PLANS FOR SPECIAL NEEDS INDIVIDUALS.—In conjunction with the periodic audit of a specialized Medicare Advantage plan for special needs individuals under paragraph (1), the Secretary shall conduct a review to ensure that such organization offering the plan meets the requirements described in section 1859(f)(5).

(e) ADDITIONAL CONTRACT TERMS.—

(1) IN GENERAL.—The contract shall contain such other terms and conditions not inconsistent with this part (including requiring the organization to provide the Secretary with such information) as the Secretary may find necessary and appropriate.

(2) COST-SHARING IN ENROLLMENT-RELATED COSTS.—

(A) IN GENERAL.—A Medicare+Choice organization and a PDP sponsor under part D shall pay the fee established by the Secretary under subparagraph (B).

(B) AUTHORIZATION.—The Secretary is authorized to charge a fee to each Medicare+Choice organization with a contract under this part and each PDP sponsor with a contract under part D that is equal to the organization' or sponsor's pro rata share (as determined by the Secretary) of the aggregate amount of fees which the Secretary is directed to collect in a fiscal year. Any amounts collected shall be available without further appropriation to the Secretary for the purpose of carrying out section 1851 (relating to enrollment and dissemination of information), section 1860D-1(c), and section 4360 of the Omnibus Budget Reconciliation Act of 1990 (relating to the health insurance counseling and assistance program).

(C) AUTHORIZATION OF APPROPRIATIONS.—There are authorized to be appropriated for the purposes described in subparagraph (B) for each fiscal year beginning with fiscal year 2001 and ending with fiscal year 2005 an amount equal to \$100,000,000, and for each fiscal year beginning with fiscal year 2006 an amount equal to \$200,000,000, reduced by the amount of fees authorized to be collected under this paragraph and section 1860D–12(b)(3)(D) for the fiscal year.

(D) LIMITATION.—In any fiscal year the fees collected by the Secretary under subparagraph (B) shall not exceed the lesser of—

(i) the estimated costs to be incurred by the Secretary in the fiscal year in carrying out the activities described in section 1851 and section 1860D–1(c) and section 4360 of the Omnibus Budget Reconciliation Act of 1990; or

(ii)(I) $200,000,000 in fiscal year 1998;

(II) $150,000,000 in fiscal year 1999;

(III) $100,000,000 in fiscal year 2000;

(IV) the Medicare+Choice portion (as defined in subparagraph (E)) of $100,000,000 in fiscal year 2001 and each succeeding fiscal year before fiscal year 2006; and

(V) the applicable portion (as defined in subparagraph (F)) of $200,000,000 in fiscal year 2006 and each succeeding fiscal year.

(E) MEDICARE+CHOICE PORTION DEFINED.—In this paragraph, the term "Medicare+Choice portion" means, for a fiscal year, the ratio, as estimated by the Secretary, of—

(i) the average number of individuals enrolled in Medicare+Choice plans during the fiscal year, to

(ii) the average number of individuals entitled to benefits under part A, and enrolled under part B, during the fiscal year.

(F) APPLICABLE PORTION DEFINED.—In this paragraph, the term "applicable portion" means, for a fiscal year—

(i) with respect to MA organizations, the Secretary's estimate of the total proportion of expenditures under this title that are attributable to expenditures made under this part (including payments under part D that are made to such organizations); or

(ii) with respect to PDP sponsors, the Secretary's estimate of the total proportion of expenditures under this title that are attributable to expenditures made to such sponsors under part D.

(3) AGREEMENTS WITH FEDERALLY QUALIFIED HEALTH CENTERS.—

(A) PAYMENT LEVELS AND AMOUNTS.—A contract under this section with an MA organization shall require the organization to provide, in any written agreement described in section 1853(a)(4) between the organization and a federally qualified health center, for a level and amount of payment to the federally qualified health center for services provided by such health center that is not less than the level and amount of payment that the plan would make for such services if the services had been furnished by a entity providing similar services that was not a federally qualified health center.

(B) COST-SHARING.—Under the written agreement reerred to in subparagraph (A), a federally qualified health center must accept the payment amount referred to in such subparagraph plus the Federal payment provided for in section 1833(a)(3)(B) as payment in full for services cov ered by the agreement, except that such a health center may collect any amount of cost-sharing permitted under the contract under this section, so long as the amounts of any deductible, coinsurance, or copayment comply with the requirements under section 1854(e).

(4) REQUIREMENT FOR MINIMUM MEDICAL LOSS RATIO.—If the Secretary determines for a contract year (beginning with 2014) that an MA plan has failed to have a medical loss ratio of at least .85—

(A) the MA plan shall remit to the Secretary an amount equal to the product of—

(i) the total revenue of the MA plan under this part for the contract year; and

(ii) the difference between .85 and the medical loss ratio;

(B) for 3 consecutive contract years, the Secretary shall not permit the enrollment of new enrollees under the plan for coverage during the second succeeding contract year; and

(C) the Secretary shall terminate the plan contract if the plan fails to have such a medical loss ratio for 5 consecutive contract years.

(5) COMMUNICATING PLAN CORRECTIVE ACTIONS AGAINST OPIOIDS OVER-PRESCRIBERS.—

(A) IN GENERAL.—Beginning with plan years beginning on or after January 1, 2021, a contract under this section with an MA organization shall require the organization to submit to the Secretary, through the process established under subparagraph (B), information on the investigations and other actions taken by such plans related to providers of services who prescribe a high volume of opioids.

(B) PROCESS.—Not later than January 1, 2021, the Secretary shall, in consultation with stakeholders, establish a process under which MA plans and prescription drug plans shall submit to the Secretary information described in subparagraph (A).

(C) REGULATIONS.—For purposes of this paragraph, including as applied under section 1860D–12(b)(3)(D), the Secretary shall, pursuant to rulemaking—

(i) specify a definition for the term "high volume of opioids" and a method for determining if a provider of services prescribes such a high volume; and

(ii) establish the process described in subparagraph

(B) and the types of information that shall be submitted through such process.

(f) PROMPT PAYMENT BY MEDICARE+CHOICE ORGANIZATION.—

(1) REQUIREMENT.—A contract under this part shall require a Medicare+Choice organization to provide prompt payment (consistent with the provisions of sections 1816(c)(2) and 1842(c)(2)) of claims submitted for services and supplies furnished to enrollees pursuant to the contract, if the services or supplies are not furnished under a contract between the organization and the provider or supplier (or in the case of a Medicare+Choice private fee-for-service plan, if a claim is submitted to such organization by an enrollee).

(2) SECRETARY'S OPTION TO BYPASS NONCOMPLYING ORGANIZATION.—In the case of a Medicare+Choice eligible organization which the Secretary determines, after notice and opportunity for a hearing, has failed to make payments of amounts in compliance with paragraph (1), the Secretary may provide for direct payment of the amounts owed to providers and suppliers (or, in the case of a Medicare+Choice private fee-for-service plan, amounts owed to the enrollees) for covered services and supplies furnished to individuals enrolled under this part under the contract. If the Secretary provides for the

direct payments, the Secretary shall provide for an appropriate reduction in the amount of payments otherwise made to the organization under this part to reflect the amount of the Secretary's payments (and the Secretary's costs in making the payments).

(3) INCORPORATION OF CERTAIN PRESCRIPTION DRUG PLAN CONTRACT REQUIREMENTS.—The following provisions shall apply to contracts with a Medicare Advantage organization offering an MA–PD plan in the same manner as they apply to contracts with a PDP sponsor offering a prescription drug plan under part D:

(A) PROMPT PAYMENT.—Section 1860D–12(b)(4).

(B) SUBMISSION OF CLAIMS BY PHARMACIES LOCATED IN OR CONTRACTING WITH LONG-TERM CARE FACILITIES.—Section 1860D–12(b)(5).

(C) REGULAR UPDATE OF PRESCRIPTION DRUG PRICING STANDARD.—Section 1860D–12(b)(6).

(g) INTERMEDIATE SANCTIONS.—

(1) IN GENERAL.—If the Secretary determines that a Medicare+Choice organization with a contract under this section—

(A) fails substantially to provide medically necessary items and services that are required (under law or under the contract) to be provided to an individual covered under the contract, if the failure has adversely affected (or has substantial likelihood of adversely affecting) the indi vidual;

(B) imposes premiums on individuals enrolled under this part in excess of the amount of the Medicare+Choice monthly basic and supplemental beneficiary premiums permitted under section 1854;

(C) acts to expel or to refuse to re-enroll an individual in violation of the provisions of this part;

(D) engages in any practice that would reasonably be expected to have the effect of denying or discouraging enrollment (except as permitted by this part) by eligible individuals with the organization whose medical condition or history indicates a need for substantial future medical serv ices;

(E) misrepresents or falsifies information that is furnished—

(i) to the Secretary under this part, or

(ii) to an individual or to any other entity under this part;

(F) fails to comply with the applicable requirements of section 1852(j)(3) or 1852(k)(2)(A)(ii);

(G) employs or contracts with any individual or entity that is excluded from participation under this title under section 1128 or 1128A for the provision of health care, utilization review, medical social work, or administrative services or employs or contracts with any entity for the provision (directly or indirectly) through such an excluded individual or entity of such services;

(H) except as provided under subparagraph (C) or (D) of section 1860D–1(b)(1), enrolls an individual in any plan under this part without the prior consent of the individual or the designee of the individual;

(I) transfers an individual enrolled under this part from one plan to another without the prior consent of the individual or the designee of the individual or solely for the purpose of earning a commission;

(J) fails to comply with marketing restrictions described in subsections (h) and (j) of section 1851 or applicable implementing regulations or guidance; or

(K) employs or contracts with any individual or entity who engages in the conduct described in subparagraphs

(A) through (J) of this paragraph;

the Secretary may provide, in addition to any other remedies authorized by law, for any of the remedies described in paragraph (2). The Secretary may provide, in addition to any other remedies authorized by law, for any of the remedies described in paragraph (2), if the Secretary determines that any employee or agent of such organization, or any provider or supplier who contracts with such organization, has engaged in any conduct described in subparagraphs (A) through (K) of this paragraph.

(2) REMEDIES.—The remedies described in this paragraph are—

(A) civil money penalties of not more than $25,000 for each determination under paragraph (1) or, with respect to a determination under subparagraph (D) or (E)(i) of such paragraph, of not more than $100,000 for each such determination, except with respect to a determination under subparagraph (E), an assessment of not more than the amount claimed by such plan or plan sponsor based upon the misrepresentation or falsified information involved, plus, with respect to a determination under paragraph (1)(B), double the excess amount charged in violation of such paragraph (and the excess amount charged shall be deducted from the penalty and returned to the individual concerned), and plus, with respect to a determination under paragraph (1)(D), $15,000 for each individual not enrolled as a result of the practice involved,

(B) suspension of enrollment of individuals under this part after the date the Secretary notifies the organization of a determination under paragraph (1) and until the Secretary is satisfied that the basis for such determination has been corrected and is not likely to recur, or

(C) suspension of payment to the organization under this part for individuals enrolled after the date the Secretary notifies the organization of a determination under paragraph (1) and until the Secretary is satisfied that the basis for such determination has been corrected and is not likely to recur.

(3) OTHER INTERMEDIATE SANCTIONS.—In the case of a Medicare+Choice organization for which the Secretary makes a determination under subsection (c)(2) the basis of which is not described in paragraph (1), the Secretary may apply the following intermediate sanctions:

(A) Civil money penalties of not more than $25,000 for each determination under subsection (c)(2) if the deficiency that is the basis of the determination has directly adversely affected (or has the substantial likelihood of adversely affecting) an individual covered under the organi zation's contract.

(B) Civil money penalties of not more than $10,000 for each week beginning after the initiation of civil money penalty procedures by the Secretary during which the deficiency that is the basis of a determination under subsection (c)(2) exists.

(C) Suspension of enrollment of individuals under this part after the date the Secretary notifies the organization of a determination under subsection (c)(2) and until the Secretary is satisfied that the deficiency that is the basis for the determination has been corrected and is not likely to recur.

(D) Civil monetary penalties of not more than $100,000, or such higher amount as the Secretary may establish by regulation, where the finding under subsection (c)(2)(A) is based on the organization's termination of its contract under this section other than at a time and in a manner provided for under subsection (a).

(4) CIVIL MONEY PENALTIES.—The provisions of section 1128A (other than subsections (a) and (b)) shall apply to a civil money penalty under paragraph (2) or (3) in the same manner as they apply to a civil money penalty or proceeding under section 1128A(a).

(h) PROCEDURES FOR TERMINATION.—

(1) IN GENERAL.—The Secretary may terminate a contract with a Medicare+Choice organization under this section in accordance with formal investigation and compliance procedures established by the Secretary under which—

(A) the Secretary provides the organization with the reasonable opportunity to develop and implement a corrective action plan to correct the deficiencies that were the basis of the Secretary's determination under subsection (c)(2); and

(B) the Secretary provides the organization with reasonable notice and opportunity for hearing (including the right to appeal an initial decision) before terminating the contract.

(2) EXCEPTION FOR IMMINENT AND SERIOUS RISK TO HEALTH.—Paragraph (1) shall not apply if the Secretary determines that a delay in termination, resulting from compliance with the procedures specified in such paragraph prior to termination, would pose an imminent and serious risk to the health of individuals enrolled under this part with the organization.

(3) DELAY IN CONTRACT TERMINATION AUTHORITY FOR PLANS FAILING TO ACHIEVE MINIMUM QUALITY RATING.—During the period beginning on the date of the enactment of this paragraph and through the end of plan year 2018, the Secretary may not terminate a contract under this section with respect to the offering of an MA plan by a

Medicare Advantage organization solely because the MA plan has failed to achieve a minimum quality rating under the 5-star rating system under section 1853(o)(4).

(i) MEDICARE+CHOICE PROGRAM COMPATIBILITY WITH EMPLOYER OR UNION GROUP HEALTH PLANS.—

(1) CONTRACTS WITH MA ORGANIZATIONS.—To facilitate the offering of Medicare+Choice plans under contracts between Medicare+Choice organizations and employers, labor organizations, or the trustees of a fund established by one or more employers or labor organizations (or combination thereof) to furnish benefits to the entity's employees, former employees (or combination thereof) or members or former members (or combination thereof) of the labor organizations, the Secretary may waive or modify requirements that hinder the design of, the offering of, or the enrollment in such Medicare+Choice plans.

(2) EMPLOYER SPONSORED MA PLANS.—To facilitate the offering of MA plans by employers, labor organizations, or the trustees of a fund established by one or more employers or labor organizations (or combination thereof) to furnish benefits to the entity's employees, former employees (or combination thereof) or members or former members (or combination thereof) of the labor organizations, the Secretary may waive or modify requirements that hinder the design of, the offering of, or the enrollment in such MA plans. Notwithstanding section 1851(g), an MA plan described in the previous sentence may restrict the enrollment of individuals under this part to individuals who are beneficiaries and participants in such plan.

## DEFINITIONS; MISCELLANEOUS PROVISIONS

SEC. 1859. (a) DEFINITIONS RELATING TO MEDICARE+CHOICE ORGANIZATIONS.—In this part—

(1) MEDICARE+CHOICE ORGANIZATION.—The term "Medicare+Choice organization" means a public or private entity that is certified under section 1856 as meeting the requirements and standards of this part for such an organization.

(2) PROVIDER-SPONSORED ORGANIZATION.—The term "provider-sponsored organization" is defined in section 1855(d)(1). (b) DEFINITIONS RELATING TO MEDICARE+CHOICE PLANS.—

(1) MEDICARE+CHOICE PLAN.—The term "Medicare+Choice plan" means health benefits coverage offered under a policy, contract, or plan by a Medicare+Choice organization pursuant to and in accordance with a contract under section 1857.

(2) MEDICARE+CHOICE PRIVATE FEE-FOR-SERVICE PLAN.—The term "Medicare+Choice private fee-for-service plan" means a Medicare+Choice plan that—

(A) reimburses hospitals, physicians, and other providers at a rate determined by the plan on a fee-for-service basis without placing the provider at financial risk;

(B) does not vary such rates for such a provider based on utilization relating to such provider; and

(C) does not restrict the selection of providers among those who are lawfully authorized to provide the covered services and agree to accept the terms and conditions of payment established by the plan.

Nothing in subparagraph (B) shall be construed to preclude a plan from varying rates for such a provider based on the spe- cialty of the provider, the location of the provider, or other fac- tors related to such provider that are not related to utilization, or to preclude a plan from increasing rates for such a provider based on increased utilization of specified preventive or screen- ing services.

(1) MSA PLAN.—

(A) IN GENERAL.—The term "MSA plan" means a Medicare+Choice plan that—

(i) provides reimbursement for at least the items and services described in section 1852(a)(1) in a year but only after the enrollee incurs countable expenses (as specified under the plan) equal to the amount of an annual deductible (described in subparagraph (B));

(ii) counts as such expenses (for purposes of such de- ductible) at least all amounts that would have been payable under parts A and B, and that would have been payable by the enrollee as deductibles, coinsur- ance, or copayments, if the enrollee had elected to re- ceive benefits through the provisions of such parts; and

(iii) provides, after such deductible is met for a year and for all subsequent expenses for items and services referred to in clause (i) in the year, for a level of reim- bursement that is not less than—

(I) 100 percent of such expenses, or

(II) 100 percent of the amounts that would have been paid (without regard to any deductibles or coinsurance) under parts A and B with respect to such expenses, whichever is less.

(B) DEDUCTIBLE.—The amount of annual deductible under an MSA plan—

(i) for contract year 1999 shall be not more than $6,000; and

(ii) for a subsequent contract year shall be not more than the maximum amount of such deductible for the previous contract year under this subparagraph increased by the national per capita Medicare+Choice growth percentage under section 1853(c)(6) for the year.

If the amount of the deductible under clause (ii) is not a multiple of $50, the amount shall be rounded to the nearest multiple of $50.

(2) MA REGIONAL PLAN.—The term "MA regional plan" means an MA plan described in section 1851(a)(2)(A)(i)—

(A) that has a network of providers that have agreed to a contractually specified reimbursement for covered benefits with the organization offering the plan;

(B) that provides for reimbursement for all covered benefits regardless of whether such benefits are provided within such network of providers; and

(C) the service area of which is one or more entire MA regions.

(3) MA LOCAL PLAN.—The term "MA local plan" means an MA plan that is not an MA regional plan.

(4) SPECIALIZED MA PLANS FOR SPECIAL NEEDS INDIVIDUALS.—

(A) IN GENERAL.—The term "specialized MA plan for special needs individuals" means an MA plan that exclusively serves special needs individuals (as defined in subparagraph (B)) and that, as of January 1,

2010, meets the applicable requirements of paragraph (2), (3), or (4) of subsection (f), as the case may be.

SPECIAL NEEDS INDIVIDUAL.—The term "special needs individual" means an MA eligible individual who—

(i) is institutionalized (as defined by the Secretary);

(ii) is entitled to medical assistance under a State plan under title XIX; or

(iii) meets such requirements as the Secretary may determine would benefit from enrollment in such a specialized MA plan described in subparagraph (A) for individuals with severe or disabling chronic conditions who—

(I) before January 1, 2022, have one or more comorbid and medically complex chronic conditions that are substantially disabling or life threatening, have a high risk of hospitalization or other significant adverse health outcomes, and require specialized delivery systems across domains of care; and

(II) on or after January 1, 2022, have one or more comorbid and medically complex chronic conditions that is life threatening or significantly limits overall health or function, have a high risk of hospitalization or other adverse health outcomes, and require intensive care coordination and that is listed under subsection (f)(9)(A).

The Secretary may apply rules similar to the rules of section 1894(c)(4) for continued eligibility of special needs individuals.

(c) OTHER REFERENCES TO OTHER TERMS.—

(1) MEDICARE+CHOICE ELIGIBLE INDIVIDUAL.—The term "Medicare+Choice eligible individual" is defined in section 1851(a)(3).

(2) MEDICARE+CHOICE PAYMENT AREA.—The term "Medicare+Choice payment area" is defined in section 1853(d).

(3) NATIONAL PER CAPITA MEDICARE+CHOICE GROWTH PERCENTAGE.—The "national per capita Medicare+Choice growth percentage" is defined in section 1853(c)(6).

(4) MEDICARE+CHOICE MONTHLY BASIC BENEFICIARY PREMIUM; MEDICARE+CHOICE MONTHLY SUPPLEMENTAL BENEFICIARY PREMIUM.—The terms "Medicare+Choice monthly

basic beneficiary premium" and "Medicare+Choice monthly supplemental beneficiary premium" are defined in section 1854(a)(2).

(5) MA LOCAL AREA.—The term "MA local area" is defined in section 1853(d)(2).

(d) COORDINATED ACUTE AND LONG-TERM CARE BENEFITS UNDER A MEDICARE+CHOICE PLAN.—Nothing in this part shall be construed as preventing a State from coordinating benefits under a medicaid plan under title XIX with those provided under a Medicare+Choice plan in a manner that assures continuity of a full-range of acute care and long-term care services to poor elderly or disabled individuals eligible for benefits under this title and under such plan.

(e) RESTRICTION ON ENROLLMENT FOR CERTAIN MEDICARE+CHOICE PLANS.—

(1) IN GENERAL.—In the case of a Medicare+Choice religious fraternal benefit society plan described in paragraph (2), not- withstanding any other provision of this part to the contrary and in accordance with regulations of the Secretary, the society offering the plan may restrict the enrollment of individuals under this part to individuals who are members of the church, convention, or group described in paragraph (3)(B) with which the society is affiliated.

(2) MEDICARE+CHOICE RELIGIOUS FRATERNAL BENEFIT SOCI- ETY PLAN DESCRIBED.—For purposes of this subsection, a Medicare+Choice religious fraternal benefit society plan de- scribed in this paragraph is a Medicare+Choice plan described in section 1851(a)(2) that—

(A) is offered by a religious fraternal benefit society de- scribed in paragraph (3) only to members of the church, convention, or group described in paragraph (3)(B); and

(B) permits all such members to enroll under the plan without regard to health status-related factors.

Nothing in this subsection shall be construed as waiving any plan requirements relating to financial solvency.

(3) RELIGIOUS FRATERNAL BENEFIT SOCIETY DEFINED.—For purposes of paragraph (2)(A), a "religious fraternal benefit society" described in this section is an organization that—

(A) is described in section 501(c)(8) of the Internal Revenue Code of 1986 and is exempt from taxation under section 501(a) of such Act;

(B) is affiliated with, carries out the tenets of, and shares a religious bond with, a church or convention or association of churches or an affiliated group of churches;

(C) offers, in addition to a Medicare+Choice religious fraternal benefit society plan, health coverage to individuals not entitled to benefits under this title who are members of such church, convention, or group; and

(D) does not impose any limitation on membership in the society based on any health status-related factor.

(4) PAYMENT ADJUSTMENT.—Under regulations of the Secretary, in the case of individuals enrolled under this part under a Medicare+Choice religious fraternal benefit society plan described in paragraph (2), the Secretary shall provide for such adjustment to the payment amounts otherwise established under section 1854 as may be appropriate to assure an appropriate payment level, taking into account the actuarial characteristics and experience of such individuals.

(f) REQUIREMENTS REGARDING ENROLLMENT IN SPECIALIZED MA PLANS FOR SPECIAL NEEDS INDIVIDUALS.—

(1) REQUIREMENTS FOR ENROLLMENT.—In the case of a specialized MA plan for special needs individuals (as defined in subsection (b)(6)), notwithstanding any other provision of this part and in accordance with regulations of the Secretary, the plan may restrict the enrollment of individuals under the plan to individuals who are within one or more classes of special needs individuals.

(2) ADDITIONAL REQUIREMENTS FOR INSTITUTIONAL SNPS.—In the case of a specialized MA plan for special needs individuals described in subsection (b)(6)(B)(i), the applicable requirements described in this paragraph are as follows:

(A) Each individual that enrolls in the plan on or after January 1, 2010, is a special needs individuals described in subsection (b)(6)(B)(i). In the case of an individual who is living in the community but requires an institutional level of care, such individual shall not be considered a special needs individual described in subsection (b)(6)(B)(i) unless the determination that the individual requires an institutional level of care was made—

(i) using a State assessment tool of the State in which the individual resides; and

(ii) by an entity other than the organization offering the plan.

(B) The plan meets the requirements described in paragraph (5).

(C) If applicable, the plan meets the requirement described in paragraph (7).

(3) ADDITIONAL REQUIREMENTS FOR DUAL SNPS.—In the case of a specialized MA plan for special needs individuals described in subsection (b)(6)(B)(ii), the applicable requirements described in this paragraph are as follows:

(A) Each individual that enrolls in the plan on or after January 1, 2010, is a special needs individuals described in subsection (b)(6)(B)(ii).

(B) The plan meets the requirements described in paragraph (5).

(C) The plan provides each prospective enrollee, prior to enrollment, with a comprehensive written statement (using standardized content and format established by the Secretary) that describes—

(i) the benefits and cost-sharing protections that the individual is entitled to under the State Medicaid program under title XIX; and

(ii) which of such benefits and cost-sharing protections are covered under the plan.

Such statement shall be included with any description of benefits offered by the plan.

(D) The plan has a contract with the State Medicaid agency to provide benefits, or arrange for benefits to be provided, for which such individual is entitled to receive as medical assistance under title XIX. Such benefits may in- clude long-term care services consistent with State policy.

(E) If applicable, the plan meets the requirement de- scribed in paragraph (7).

(F) The plan meets the requirements applicable under paragraph (8).

(4) ADDITIONAL REQUIREMENTS FOR SEVERE OR DISABLING CHRONIC CONDITION SNPS.—In the case of a specialized MA plan for special needs individuals described in subsection (b)(6)(B)(iii), the applicable requirements described in this paragraph are as follows:

(A) Each individual that enrolls in the plan on or after January 1, 2010, is a special needs individual described in subsection (b)(6)(B)(iii).

(B) The plan meets the requirements described in paragraph (5).

(C) If applicable, the plan meets the requirement described in paragraph (7).

(5) CARE MANAGEMENT REQUIREMENTS FOR ALL SNPS.—

(A) IN GENERAL.—Subject to subparagraph (B), the requirements described in this paragraph are that the organization offering a specialized MA plan for special needs individuals—

(i) have in place an evidenced-based model of care with appropriate networks of providers and specialists; and

(ii) with respect to each individual enrolled in the plan—

(I) conduct an initial assessment and an annual reassessment of the individual's physical, psychosocial, and functional needs;

(II) develop a plan, in consultation with the individual as feasible, that identifies goals and objectives, including measurable outcomes as well as specific services and benefits to be provided; and

(III) use an interdisciplinary team in the management of care.

(B) IMPROVEMENTS TO CARE MANAGEMENT REQUIREMENTS FOR SEVERE OR DISABLING CHRONIC CONDITION SNPS.—For 2020 and subsequent years, in the case of a specialized MA plan for special needs individuals described in subsection (b)(6)(B)(iii), the requirements described in this paragraph include the following:

(i) The interdisciplinary team under subparagraph (A)(ii)(III) includes a team of providers with demonstrated expertise, including training in an applicable specialty, in treating individuals similar to the targeted population of the plan.

(ii) Requirements developed by the Secretary to provide face-to-face encounters with individuals enrolled in the plan not less frequently than on an annual basis.

(III) As part of the model of care under clause (i) of subparagraph (A), the results of the initial assessment and annual reassessment under clause (ii)(I) of such subparagraph of each individual enrolled in the plan are addressed in the individual's individualized care plan under clause (ii)(II) of such subparagraph.

(iv) As part of the annual evaluation and approval of such model of care, the Secretary shall take into account whether the plan fulfilled the previous year's goals (as required under the model of care).

(v) The Secretary shall establish a minimum benchmark for each element of the model of care of a plan. The Secretary shall only approve a plan's model of care under this paragraph if each element of the model of care meets the minimum benchmark applicable under the preceding sentence.

(6) TRANSITION AND EXCEPTION REGARDING RESTRICTION ON ENROLLMENT.—

(A) IN GENERAL.—Subject to subparagraph (C), the Secretary shall establish procedures for the transition of applicable individuals to—

(i) a Medicare Advantage plan that is not a specialized MA plan for special needs individuals (as defined in subsection (b)(6)); or

(ii) the original medicare fee-for-service program under parts A and B.

(B) APPLICABLE INDIVIDUALS.—For purposes of clause (i), the term "applicable individual" means an individual who—

(i) is enrolled under a specialized MA plan for special needs individuals (as defined in subsection (b)(6)); and

(ii) is not within the 1 or more of the classes of special needs individuals to which enrollment under the plan is restricted to.

(C) EXCEPTION.—The Secretary shall provide for an exception to the transition described in subparagraph (A) for a limited period of time for individuals enrolled under a specialized MA plan for special needs individuals described in subsection (b)(6)(B)(ii) who are no longer eligible for medical assistance under title XIX.

(D) TIMELINE FOR INITIAL TRANSITION.—The Secretary shall ensure that applicable individuals enrolled in a specialized MA plan for special needs individuals (as defined in subsection (b)(6)) prior to January 1, 2010, are transitioned to a plan or the program described in subparagraph (A) by not later than January 1, 2013.

(7) AUTHORITY TO REQUIRE SPECIAL NEEDS PLANS BE NCQA APPROVED.—For 2012 and subsequent years, the Secretary shall require that a Medicare Advantage organization offering a specialized MA plan for special needs individuals be approved by the National Committee for Quality Assurance (based on standards established by the Secretary).

(8) INCREASED INTEGRATION OF DUAL SNPS.—

(A) DESIGNATED CONTACT.—The Secretary, acting through the Federal Coordinated Health Care Office established under section 2602 of Public Law 111–148, shall serve as a dedicated point of contact for States to address misalignments that arise with the integration of specialized MA plans for special needs individuals described in subsection (b)(6)(B)(ii) under this paragraph and, consistent with such role, shall establish—

(i) a uniform process for disseminating to State Medicaid agencies information under this title impacting contracts between such agencies and such plans under this subsection; and

(ii) basic resources for States interested in exploring such plans as a platform for integration, such as a model contract or other tools to achieve those goals.

(B) UNIFIED GRIEVANCES AND APPEALS PROCESS.—

(i) IN GENERAL.—Not later than April 1, 2020, the Secretary shall establish procedures, to the extent feasible as determined by the Secretary, unifying grievances and appeals procedures under sections 1852(f), 1852(g), 1902(a)(3), 1902(a)(5), and 1932(b)(4) for items and services provided by specialized MA plans for special needs individuals described in subsection (b)(6)(B)(ii) under this title and title XIX. With respect to items and services described in the preceding sentence, procedures established under this clause shall apply in place of otherwise applicable grievances and appeals procedures. The Secretary shall solicit comment in developing such procedures from States, plans, beneficiaries and their representatives, and other relevant stakeholders.

(ii) PROCEDURES.—The procedures established under clause (i) shall be included in the plan contract under paragraph (3)(D) and shall—

(I) adopt the provisions for the enrollee that are most protective for the enrollee and, to the extent feasible as determined by the Secretary, are compatible with unified timeframes and consolidated access to external review under an integrated process;

(II) take into account differences in State plans under title XIX to the extent necessary;

(III) be easily navigable by an enrollee; and

(IV) include the elements described in clause (iii), as applicable.

(iii) ELEMENTS DESCRIBED.—Both unified appeals and unified grievance procedures shall include, as applicable, the following elements described in this clause:

(I) Single written notification of all applicable grievances and appeal rights under this title and title XIX. For purposes of this subparagraph, the Secretary may waive the requirements under section 1852(g)(1)(B) when the specialized MA plan covers items or services under this part or under title XIX.

(II) Single pathways for resolution of any grievance or appeal related to a particular item or service provided by specialized MA plans for special needs individuals described in subsection (b)(6)(B)(ii) under this title and title XIX.

(III) Notices written in plain language and available in a language and format that is accessible to the enrollee, including in non-English languages that are prevalent in the service area of the specialized MA plan.

(IV) Unified timeframes for grievances and appeals processes, such as an individual's filing of a grievance or appeal, a plan's acknowledgment and resolution of a grievance or appeal, and notification of decisions with respect to a grievance or appeal.

(V) Requirements for how the plan must process, track, and resolve grievances and appeals, to ensure beneficiaries are notified on a timely basis of decisions that are made throughout the grievance or appeals process and are able to easily determine the status of a grievance or appeal.

(iv) CONTINUATION OF BENEFITS PENDING APPEAL.— The unified procedures under clause (i) shall, with respect to all benefits under parts A and B and title XIX subject to appeal under such procedures, incorporate provisions under current law and implementing regulations that provide continuation of benefits pending appeal under this title and title XIX.

(C) REQUIREMENT FOR UNIFIED GRIEVANCES AND APPEALS.—For 2021 and subsequent years, the contract of a specialized MA plan for special needs individuals described in subsection (b)(6)(B)(ii) with a State Medicaid agency under paragraph (3)(D) shall require the use of unified grievances and appeals procedures as described in subparagraph (B).

(D) REQUIREMENTS FOR INTEGRATION.—

(i) IN GENERAL.—For 2021 and subsequent years, a specialized MA plan for special needs individuals described in subsection (b)(6)(B)(ii) shall meet one or more of the following requirements, to the extent permitted under State law, for integration of benefits under this title and title XIX:

(I) The specialized MA plan must meet the requirements of contracting with the State Medicaid agency described in paragraph (3)(D) in addition to coordinating long-term services and supports or behavioral health services, or both, by meeting an additional minimum set of requirements determined by the Secretary through the Federal Coordinated Health Care Office established under section 2602 of the Patient Protection and Affordable Care Act based on input from stakeholders, such as notifying the State in a timely manner of hospitalizations, emergency room visits, and hospital or nursing home discharges of enrollees, assigning one primary care provider for each enrollee, or sharing data that would benefit the coordination of items and services under this title and the State plan under title XIX. Such minimum set of requirements must be included in the contract of the specialized MA plan with the State Medicaid agency under such paragraph.

(II) The specialized MA plan must meet the requirements of a fully integrated plan described in section 1853(a)(1)(B)(iv)(II) (other than the requirement that the plan have similar average levels of frailty, as determined by the Secretary, as the PACE program), or enter into a capitated contract with the State Medicaid agency to provide long-term services and supports or behavioral health services, or both.

(III) In the case of a specialized MA plan that is offered by a parent organization that is also the parent organization of a Medicaid managed care organization providing long term services and supports or behavioral services under a contract under section 1903(m), the parent organization must assume clinical and financial responsibility for benefits provided under this title and title XIX with respect to any individual who is enrolled in both the specialized MA plan and the Medicaid managed care organization.

(ii) SUSPENSION OF ENROLLMENT FOR FAILURE TO MEET REQUIREMENTS DURING INITIAL PERIOD.—During the period of plan years 2021 through 2025, if the Secretary determines that a specialized MA plan for special needs individuals described in subsection (b)(6)(B)(ii) has failed to comply with clause (i), the Secretary may provide for the application against the Medicare Advantage organization offering the plan of the remedy described in section 1857(g)(2)(B) in the same manner as the Secretary may apply such remedy, and in accordance with the same procedures as would apply, in the case of an MA organization determined by the Secretary to have engaged in conduct described in section 1857(g)(1). If the Secretary applies such remedy to a Medicare Advantage organization under the preceding sentence, the organization shall submit to the Secretary (at a time, and in a form and manner, specified by the Secretary) information describing how the plan will come into compliance with clause (i).

(E) STUDY AND REPORT TO CONGRESS.—

(i) IN GENERAL.—Not later than March 15, 2022, and, subject to clause (iii), biennially thereafter through 2032, the Medicare Payment Advisory Commission established under section 1805, in consultation with the Medicaid and CHIP Payment and Access Commission established under section 1900, shall conduct (and submit to the Secretary and the Committees on Ways and Means and Energy and Commerce of the House of Representatives and the Committee on Finance of the Senate a report on) a study to determine how specialized MA plans for special needs individuals described in subsection (b)(6)(B)(ii) perform among each other based on data from Healthcare Effectiveness Data and Information Set (HEDIS) quality measures, reported on the plan level, as required under section 1852(e)(3) (or such other measures or data sources that are available and appropriate, such as encounter data and Consumer Assessment of Healthcare Providers and Systems data, as specified by such Commissions as enabling an accurate evaluation under this subparagraph). Such study shall include, as feasible, the following comparison groups of specialized MA plans for special needs individuals described in subsection (b)(6)(B)(ii):

(I) A comparison group of such plans that are described in subparagraph (D)(i)(I).

(II) A comparison group of such plans that are described in subparagraph (D)(i)(II).

(III) A comparison group of such plans operating within the Financial Alignment Initiative demonstration for the period for which such plan is so operating and the demonstration is in effect, and, in the case that an integration option that is not with respect to specialized MA plans for special needs individuals is established after the conclusion of the demonstration involved.

(IV) A comparison group of such plans that are described in subparagraph (D)(i)(III).

(V) A comparison group of MA plans, as feasible, not described in a previous subclause of this clause, with respect to the performance of such plans for enrollees who are special needs individuals described in subsection (b)(6)(B)(ii).

(ii) ADDITIONAL REPORTS.—Beginning with 2033 and every five years thereafter, the Medicare Payment Advisory Commission, in consultation with the Medicaid and CHIP Payment and Access Commission, shall conduct a study described in clause (i).

(9) LIST OF CONDITIONS FOR CLARIFICATION OF THE DEFINITION OF A SEVERE OR DISABLING CHRONIC CONDITIONS SPECIALIZED NEEDS INDIVIDUAL.—

(A) IN GENERAL.—Not later than December 31, 2020, and every 5 years thereafter, subject to subparagraphs (B) and (C), the Secretary shall convene a panel of clinical advisors to establish and update a list of conditions that meet each of the following criteria:

(i) Conditions that meet the definition of a severe or disabling chronic condition under subsection (b)(6)(B)(iii) on or after January 1, 2022.

(ii) Conditions that require prescription drugs, providers, and models of care that are unique to the specific population of enrollees in a specialized MA plan for special needs individuals described in such subsection on or after such date and—

(I) as a result of access to, and enrollment in, such a specialized MA plan for special needs individuals, individuals with such condition would have a reasonable expectation of slowing or halting the progression of the disease, improving health outcomes and decreasing overall costs for individuals diagnosed with such condition compared to available options of care other than through such a specialized MA plan for special needs individuals; or

(II) have a low prevalence in the general population of beneficiaries under this title or a disproportionally high per-beneficiary cost under this title.

(B) INCLUSION OF CERTAIN CONDITIONS.—The conditions listed under subparagraph (A) shall include HIV/AIDS, end stage renal disease, and chronic and disabling mental illness.

(C) REQUIREMENT.—In establishing and updating the list under subparagraph (A), the panel shall take into account the availability of varied benefits, cost-sharing, and supplemental benefits under the model described in paragraph (2) of section 1859(h), including the expansion under paragraph (1) of such section.

(g) SPECIAL RULES FOR SENIOR HOUSING FACILITY PLANS.—

(1) IN GENERAL.—In the case of a Medicare Advantage senior housing facility plan described in paragraph (2), notwithstanding any other provision of this part to the contrary and in accordance with regulations of the Secretary, the service area of such plan may be limited to a senior housing facility in a geographic area.

(2) MEDICARE ADVANTAGE SENIOR HOUSING FACILITY PLAN DESCRIBED.—For purposes of this subsection, a Medicare Advantage senior housing facility plan is a Medicare Advantage plan that—

(A) restricts enrollment of individuals under this part to individuals who reside in a continuing care retirement community (as defined in section 1852(l)(4)(B));

(B) provides primary care services onsite and has a ratio of accessible physicians to beneficiaries that the Secretary determines is adequate;

(C) provides transportation services for beneficiaries to specialty providers outside of the facility; and

(D) has participated (as of December 31, 2009) in a demonstration project established by the Secretary under which such a plan was offered for not less than 1 year.

(h) NATIONAL TESTING OF MEDICARE ADVANTAGE VALUE-BASED INSURANCE DESIGN MODEL.—

(1) IN GENERAL.—In implementing the Medicare Advantage Value-Based Insurance Design model that is being tested under section 1115A(b), the Secretary shall revise the testing of the model under such section to cover, effective not later than January 1, 2020, all States.

(2) TERMINATION AND MODIFICATION PROVISION NOT APPLICABLE UNTIL JANUARY 1, 2022.—The provisions of section 1115A(b)(3)(B) shall apply to the Medicare Advantage Value-Based Insurance Design model, including such model as revised under paragraph (1), beginning January 1, 2022, but shall not apply to such model, as so revised, prior to such date.

(3) FUNDING.—The Secretary shall allocate funds made available under section 1115A(f)(1) to design, implement, and evaluate the Medicare

Advantage Value-Based Insurance Design model, as revised under paragraph (1).

(i) PROGRAM INTEGRITY TRANSPARENCY MEASURES.—

(1) PROGRAM INTEGRITY PORTAL.—

(A) IN GENERAL.—Not later than two years after the date of the enactment of this subsection, the Secretary shall, after consultation with stakeholders, establish a secure Internet website portal (or other successor technology) that would allow a secure path for communication between the Secretary, MA plans under this part, prescription drug plans under part D, and an eligible entity with a contract under section 1893 (such as a Medicare drug integrity contractor or an entity responsible for carrying out program integrity activities under this part and part D) for the purpose of enabling through such portal (or other successor technology)—

(i) the referral by such plans of substantiated fraud, waste, and abuse for initiating or assisting investigations conducted by the eligible entity; and

(ii) data sharing among such MA plans, prescription drug plans, and the Secretary.

(B) REQUIRED USES OF PORTAL.—The Secretary shall disseminate the following information to MA plans under this part and prescription drug plans under part D through the secure Internet website portal (or other successor technology) established under subparagraph (A):

(i) Providers of services and suppliers that have been referred pursuant to subparagraph (A)(i) during the previous 12-month period.

(ii) Providers of services and suppliers who are the subject of an active exclusion under section 1128 or who are subject to a suspension of payment under this title pursuant to section 1862(o) or otherwise.

(iii) Providers of services and suppliers who are the subject of an active revocation of participation under this title, including for not satisfying conditions of participation.

(iv) In the case of such a plan that makes a referral under subparagraph (A)(i) through the portal (or other successor technology) with respect to activities of substantiated fraud, waste, or abuse of a provider of services or supplier, if such provider or supplier has been the subject of an administrative action under this title or title XI with respect to similar activities, a notification to such plan of such action so taken.

(C) RULEMAKING.—For purposes of this paragraph, the Secretary shall, through rulemaking, specify what constitutes substantiated fraud, waste, and abuse, using guidance such as what is provided in the Medicare Program Integrity Manual 4.7.1. In carrying out the previous sentence, for purposes of this paragraph, a fraud hotline tip (as defined by the Secretary) without further evidence shall not be treated as sufficient evidence for substantiated fraud, waste, or abuse.

(D) HIPAA COMPLIANT INFORMATION ONLY.—For purposes of this subsection, communications may only occur if the communications are permitted under the Federal regulations (concerning the privacy of individually identifiable health information) promulgated under section 264(c) of the Health Insurance Portability and Accountability Act of 1996.

(2) QUARTERLY REPORTS.—Beginning two years after the date of enactment of this subsection, the Secretary shall make available to MA plans under this part and prescription drug plans under part D in a timely manner (but no less frequently than quarterly) and using information submitted to an entity described in paragraph (1) through the portal (or other successor technology) described in such paragraph or pursuant to section 1893, information on fraud, waste, and abuse schemes and trends in identifying suspicious activity. Information included in each such report shall—

(A) include administrative actions, pertinent information related to opioid overprescribing, and other data determined appropriate by the Secretary in consultation with stakeholders; and

(B) be anonymized information submitted by plans without identifying the source of such information.

(3) CLARIFICATION.—Nothing in this subsection shall be construed as precluding or otherwise affecting referrals described in subparagraph (A) that may otherwise be made to law enforcement entities or to the Secretary.

PART D—Voluntary Prescription Drug Benefit Program. Subpart 1—Part D Eligible Individuals And Prescription Drug Benefits. Beneficiary Protections For Qualified Prescription Drug Coverage.

SEC. 1860D–4. (a) DISSEMINATION OF INFORMATION.—

(1) GENERAL INFORMATION.—

(A) APPLICATION OF MA INFORMATION.—A PDP sponsor shall disclose, in a clear, accurate, and standardized form to each enrollee with a prescription drug plan offered by the sponsor under this part at the time of enrollment and at least annually thereafter, the information described in section 1852(c)(1) relating to such plan, insofar as the Secretary determines appropriate with respect to benefits provided under this part, and including the information described in subparagraph (B).

(B) DRUG SPECIFIC INFORMATION.—The information described in this subparagraph is information concerning the following:

(i) Access to specific covered part D drugs, including access through pharmacy networks.

(ii) How any formulary (including any tiered formulary structure) used by the sponsor functions, including a description of how a part D eligible individual may obtain information on the formulary consistent with paragraph (3).

(iii) Beneficiary cost-sharing requirements and how a part D eligible individual may obtain information on such requirements, including tiered or other copayment level applicable to each drug (or class of drugs), consistent with paragraph (3).

(iv) The medication therapy management program required under subsection (c).

(v) The drug management program for at-risk beneficiaries under subsection (c)(5).

(2) DISCLOSURE UPON REQUEST OF GENERAL COVERAGE, UTILIZATION, AND GRIEVANCE INFORMATION.—Upon request of a part D eligible individual who is eligible to enroll in a prescription drug plan, the PDP sponsor offering such plan shall provide information similar (as determined by the Secretary) to the information described in subparagraphs (A), (B), and (C) of section 1852(c)(2) to such individual.

(3) PROVISION OF SPECIFIC INFORMATION.—

(A) RESPONSE TO BENEFICIARY QUESTIONS.—Each PDP sponsor offering a prescription drug plan shall have a mechanism for providing specific information on a timely basis to enrollees upon request. Such mechanism shall include access to information through the use of a toll-free telephone number and, upon request, the provision of such information in writing.

(B) AVAILABILITY OF INFORMATION ON CHANGES IN FORMULARY THROUGH THE INTERNET.—A PDP sponsor offering a prescription drug plan shall make available on a timely basis through an Internet website information on specific changes in the formulary under the plan (including changes to tiered or preferred status of covered part D drugs).

(4) CLAIMS INFORMATION.—A PDP sponsor offering a prescription drug plan must furnish to each enrollee in a form easily understandable to such enrollees—

(A) an explanation of benefits (in accordance with section 1806(a) or in a comparable manner); and

(B) when prescription drug benefits are provided under this part, a notice of the benefits in relation to—

(i) the initial coverage limit for the current year; and

(ii) the annual out-of-pocket threshold for the current year.

Notices under subparagraph (B) need not be provided more often than as specified by the Secretary and notices under subparagraph (B)(ii) shall take into account the application of section 1860D–2(b)(4)(C) to the extent practicable, as specified by the Secretary.

(b) ACCESS TO COVERED PART D DRUGS.—

(1) ASSURING PHARMACY ACCESS.—

(A) PARTICIPATION OF ANY WILLING PHARMACY.—A prescription drug plan shall permit the participation of any pharmacy that meets the terms and conditions under the plan.

(B) DISCOUNTS ALLOWED FOR NETWORK PHARMACIES.—For covered part D drugs dispensed through in-network pharmacies, a prescription drug plan may, notwithstanding subparagraph (A), reduce coinsurance or copayments for part D eligible individuals enrolled in the plan below the level otherwise required. In no case shall such a reduction result in an increase in payments made by the Secretary under section 1860D–15 to a plan.

(C) CONVENIENT ACCESS FOR NETWORK PHARMACIES.—

(i) IN GENERAL.—The PDP sponsor of the prescription drug plan shall secure the participation in its network of a sufficient number of pharmacies that dispense (other than by mail order) drugs directly to patients to ensure convenient access (consistent with rules established by the Secretary).

(ii) APPLICATION OF TRICARE STANDARDS.—The Secretary shall establish rules for convenient access to innetwork pharmacies under this subparagraph that are no less favorable to enrollees than the rules for convenient access to pharmacies included in the statement of work of solicitation (#MDA906–03–R–0002) of the Department of Defense under the TRICARE Retail Pharmacy (TRRx) as of March 13, 2003.

(iii) ADEQUATE EMERGENCY ACCESS.—Such rules shall include adequate emergency access for enrollees.

(iv) CONVENIENT ACCESS IN LONG-TERM CARE FACILITIES.—Such rules may include standards with respect to access for enrollees who are residing in long-term care facilities and for pharmacies operated by the Indian Health Service, Indian tribes and tribal organizations, and urban Indian organizations (as defined in section 4 of the Indian Health Care Improvement Act).

(D) LEVEL PLAYING FIELD.—Such a sponsor shall permit enrollees to receive benefits (which may include a 90-day supply of drugs or biologicals) through a pharmacy (other than a mail order pharmacy), with any differential in charge paid by such enrollees.

(E) NOT REQUIRED TO ACCEPT INSURANCE RISK.—The terms and conditions under subparagraph (A) may not require participating pharmacies to accept insurance risk as a condition of participation.

(2) USE OF STANDARDIZED TECHNOLOGY.—

(A) IN GENERAL.—The PDP sponsor of a prescription drug plan shall issue (and reissue, as appropriate) such a card (or other technology) that may be used by an enrollee to assure access to negotiated prices under section 1860D– 2(d).

(B) STANDARDS.—

(i) IN GENERAL.—The Secretary shall provide for the development, adoption, or recognition of standards relating to a standardized format for the card or other technology required under subparagraph (A). Such standards shall be compatible with part C of title XI and may be based on standards developed by an appropriate standard setting organization.

(ii) CONSULTATION.—In developing the standards under clause (i), the Secretary shall consult with the National Council for Prescription Drug Programs and other standard setting organizations determined appropriate by the Secretary.

(iii) IMPLEMENTATION.—The Secretary shall develop, adopt, or recognize the standards under clause (i) by such date as the Secretary determines shall be sufficient to ensure that PDP sponsors utilize such standards beginning January 1, 2006.

(3) REQUIREMENTS ON DEVELOPMENT AND APPLICATION OF FORMULARIES.—If a PDP sponsor of a prescription drug plan uses a formulary (including the use of tiered cost-sharing), the following requirements must be met:

(A) DEVELOPMENT AND REVISION BY A PHARMACY AND THERAPEUTIC (P&T) COMMITTEE.—

(i) IN GENERAL.—The formulary must be developed and reviewed by a pharmacy and therapeutic committee. A majority of the members of such committee

shall consist of individuals who are practicing physicians or practicing pharmacists (or both).

(ii) INCLUSION OF INDEPENDENT EXPERTS.—Such committee shall include at least one practicing physician and at least one practicing pharmacist, each of whom—

(I) is independent and free of conflict with respect to the sponsor and plan; and

(II) has expertise in the care of elderly or disabled persons.

(B) FORMULARY DEVELOPMENT.—In developing and reviewing the formulary, the committee shall—

(i) base clinical decisions on the strength of scientific evidence and standards of practice, including assessing peer-reviewed medical literature, such as randomized clinical trials, pharmacoeconomic studies, outcomes research data, and on such other information as the committee determines to be appropriate; and

(ii) take into account whether including in the formulary (or in a tier in such formulary) particular covered part D drugs has therapeutic advantages in terms of safety and efficacy.

(C) INCLUSION OF DRUGS IN ALL THERAPEUTIC CATEGORIES AND CLASSES.—

(i) IN GENERAL.—Subject to subparagraph (G), the formulary must include drugs within each therapeutic category and class of covered part D drugs, although not necessarily all drugs within such categories and classes.

(ii) MODEL GUIDELINES.—The Secretary shall request the United States Pharmacopeia to develop, in consultation with pharmaceutical benefit managers and other interested parties, a list of categories and classes that may be used by prescription drug plans under this paragraph and to revise such classification from time to time to reflect changes in therapeutic uses of covered part D drugs and the additions of new covered part D drugs.

(iii) LIMITATION ON CHANGES IN THERAPEUTIC CLASSIFICATION.—The PDP sponsor of a prescription drug plan may not change the therapeutic categories and classes in a formulary other than at the beginning of each plan year except as the Secretary may permit to take into account new therapeutic uses and newly approved covered part D drugs.

(D) PROVIDER AND PATIENT EDUCATION.—The PDP sponsor shall establish policies and procedures to educate and inform health care providers and enrollees concerning the formulary.

(E) NOTICE BEFORE REMOVING DRUG FROM FORMULARY OR CHANGING PREFERRED OR TIER STATUS OF DRUG.—Any removal of a covered part D drug from a formulary and any change in the preferred or tiered cost-sharing status of such a drug shall take effect only after appropriate no- tice is made available (such as under subsection (a)(3)) to the Secretary, affected enrollees, physicians, pharmacies, and pharmacists.

(F) PERIODIC EVALUATION OF PROTOCOLS.—In connection with the formulary, the sponsor of a prescription drug plan shall provide for the periodic evaluation and analysis of treatment protocols and procedures.

(G) REQUIRED INCLUSION OF DRUGS IN CERTAIN CATEGORIES AND CLASSES.—

(i) FORMULARY REQUIREMENTS.—

(I) IN GENERAL.—Subject to subclause (II), a PDP sponsor offering a prescription drug plan shall be required to include all covered part D drugs in the categories and classes identified by the Secretary under clause (ii)(I).

(II) EXCEPTIONS.—The Secretary may establish exceptions that permit a PDP sponsor offering a prescription drug plan to exclude from its formulary a particular covered part D drug in a category or class that is otherwise required to be included in the formulary under subclause (I) (or to otherwise limit access to such a drug, including through prior authorization or utilization management).

(ii) IDENTIFICATION OF DRUGS IN CERTAIN CATEGORIES AND CLASSES.—

(I) IN GENERAL.—Subject to clause (iv), the Secretary shall identify, as appropriate, categories and classes of drugs for which the Secretary determines are of clinical concern.

(II) CRITERIA.—The Secretary shall use criteria established by the Secretary in making any determination under subclause (I).

(iii) IMPLEMENTATION.—The Secretary shall establish the criteria under clause (ii)(II) and any exceptions under clause (i)(II) through the promulgation of a regulation which includes a public notice and comment period.

(iv) REQUIREMENT FOR CERTAIN CATEGORIES AND CLASSES UNTIL CRITERIA ESTABLISHED.—Until such time as the Secretary establishes the criteria under clause (ii)(II) the following categories and classes of drugs shall be identified under clause (ii)(I):

(I) Anticonvulsants.

(II) Antidepressants.

(III) Antineoplastics.

(IV) Antipsychotics.

(V) Antiretrovirals.

(VI) Immunosuppressants for the treatment of transplant rejection.

(H) USE OF SINGLE, UNIFORM EXCEPTIONS AND APPEALS PROCESS.—Notwithstanding any other provision of this part, each PDP sponsor of a prescription drug plan shall—

(i) use a single, uniform exceptions and appeals process (including, to the extent the Secretary determines feasible, a single, uniform model form for use under such process) with respect to the determination of prescription drug coverage for an enrollee under the plan; and

(ii) provide instant access to such process by enrollees through a toll-free telephone number and an Internet website.

(c) COST AND UTILIZATION MANAGEMENT; QUALITY ASSURANCE; MEDICATION THERAPY MANAGEMENT PROGRAM.—

(1) IN GENERAL.—The PDP sponsor shall have in place, directly or through appropriate arrangements, with respect to covered part D drugs, the following:

(A) A cost-effective drug utilization management program, including incentives to reduce costs when medically appropriate, such as through the use of multiple source drugs (as defined in section 1927(k)(7)(A)(i)).

(B) Quality assurance measures and systems to reduce medication errors and adverse drug interactions and improve medication use.

(C) A medication therapy management program described in paragraph (2).

(D) A program to control fraud, abuse, and waste.

(E) A utilization management tool to prevent drug abuse (as described in paragraph (6)(A)).

Nothing in this section shall be construed as impairing a PDP sponsor from utilizing cost management tools (including differential payments) under all methods of operation.

(2) MEDICATION THERAPY MANAGEMENT PROGRAM.—

(A) DESCRIPTION.—

(i) IN GENERAL.—A medication therapy management program described in this paragraph is a program of drug therapy management that may be furnished by a pharmacist and that is designed to assure, with respect to targeted beneficiaries described in clause (ii), that covered part D drugs under the prescription drug plan are appropriately used to optimize therapeutic outcomes through improved medication use, and to reduce the risk of adverse events, including adverse drug interactions. Such a program may distinguish between services in ambulatory and institutional settings.

(ii) TARGETED BENEFICIARIES DESCRIBED.—Targeted beneficiaries described in this clause are part D eligible individuals who—

(I) have multiple chronic diseases (such as diabetes, asthma, hypertension, hyperlipidemia, and congestive heart failure);

(II) are taking multiple covered part D drugs; and

(III) are identified as likely to incur annual costs for covered part D drugs that exceed a level specified by the Secretary.

(B) ELEMENTS.—Such program may include elements that promote—

(i) enhanced enrollee understanding to promote the appropriate use of medications by enrollees and to reduce the risk of potential adverse events associated with medications, through beneficiary education, counseling, and other appropriate means;

(ii) increased enrollee adherence with prescription medication regimens through medication refill reminders, special packaging, and other compliance programs and other appropriate means; and

(iii) detection of adverse drug events and patterns of overuse and underuse of prescription drugs.

(C) REQUIRED INTERVENTIONS.—For plan years beginning on or after the date that is 2 years after the date of the enactment of the Patient Protection and Affordable Care Act, prescription drug plan sponsors shall offer medication therapy management services to targeted beneficiaries described in subparagraph (A)(ii) that include, at a minimum, the following to increase adherence to prescription medications or other goals deemed necessary by the Secretary:

(i) An annual comprehensive medication review furnished person-to-person or using telehealth technologies (as defined by the Secretary) by a licensed pharmacist or other qualified provider. The comprehensive medication review—

(I) shall include a review of the individual's medications and may result in the creation of a recommended medication action plan or other actions in consultation with the individual and with input from the prescriber to the extent necessary and practicable; and

(II) shall include providing the individual with a written or printed summary of the results of the review.

The Secretary, in consultation with relevant stakeholders, shall develop a standardized format for the action plan under subclause (I) and the summary under subclause (II).

(ii) Follow-up interventions as warranted based on the findings of the annual medication review or the targeted medication enrollment and which may be provided person-to-person or using telehealth technologies (as defined by the Secretary).

(D) ASSESSMENT.—The prescription drug plan sponsor shall have in place a process to assess, at least on a quarterly basis, the medication use of individuals who are at risk but not enrolled in the medication therapy management program, including individuals who have experienced a transition in care, if the prescription drug plan sponsor has access to that information.

(E) AUTOMATIC ENROLLMENT WITH ABILITY TO OPT-OUT.— The prescription drug plan sponsor shall have in place a process to—

(i) subject to clause (ii), automatically enroll targeted beneficiaries described in subparagraph (A)(ii), including beneficiaries identified under subparagraph (D), in the medication therapy management program required under this subsection; and

(ii) permit such beneficiaries to opt-out of enrollment in such program.

(E) DEVELOPMENT OF PROGRAM IN COOPERATION WITH LICENSED PHARMACISTS.—Such program shall be developed in cooperation with licensed and practicing pharmacists and physicians.

(F) COORDINATION WITH CARE MANAGEMENT PLANS.—The Secretary shall establish guidelines for the coordination of any medication therapy management program under this paragraph with respect to a targeted beneficiary with any care management plan established with respect to such beneficiary under a chronic care improvement program under section 1807.

(G) CONSIDERATIONS IN PHARMACY FEES.—The PDP sponsor of a prescription drug plan shall take into account, in establishing fees for pharmacists and others providing services under such plan, the resources used, and time required to, implement the medication therapy management program under this paragraph. Each such sponsor shall disclose to the Secretary upon request the amount of any such management or dispensing fees. The provisions of section 1927(b)(3)(D) apply to information disclosed under this subparagraph.

(3) REDUCING WASTEFUL DISPENSING OF OUTPATIENT PRESCRIPTION DRUGS IN LONG-TERM CARE FACILITIES.—The Secretary shall require PDP sponsors of prescription drug plans to utilize specific, uniform dispensing techniques, as determined by the Secretary, in consultation with relevant stakeholders (including representatives of nursing facilities, residents of nursing facilities, pharmacists, the pharmacy industry (including retail and long-term care pharmacy), prescription drug plans, MA–PD plans, and any other stakeholders the Secretary determines appropriate), such as weekly, daily, or automated dose dispensing, when dispensing covered part D drugs to enrollees who reside in a long-term care facility in order to reduce waste associated with 30-day fills.

(4) REQUIRING VALID PRESCRIBER NATIONAL PROVIDER IDENTIFIERS ON PHARMACY CLAIMS.—

(A) IN GENERAL.—For plan year 2016 and subsequent plan years, the Secretary shall require a claim for a covered part D drug for a part D eligible individual enrolled in a prescription drug plan under this part or an MA–PD plan under part C to include a prescriber National Provider Identifier that is determined to be valid under the procedures established under subparagraph (B)(i).

(B) PROCEDURES.—

(i) VALIDITY OF PRESCRIBER NATIONAL PROVIDER IDENTIFIERS.—The Secretary, in consultation with appropriate stakeholders, shall establish procedures for determining the validity of prescriber National Provider Identifiers under subparagraph (A).

(ii) INFORMING BENEFICIARIES OF REASON FOR DENIAL.—The Secretary shall establish procedures to ensure that, in the case that a claim for a covered part D drug of an individual described in subparagraph (A) is denied because the claim does not meet the requirements of this paragraph, the individual is properly informed at the point of service of the reason for the denial.

REPORT.—Not later than January 1, 2018, the Inspector General of the Department of Health and Human Services shall submit to Congress a report on the effectiveness of the procedures established under subparagraph (B)(i).

(5) DRUG MANAGEMENT PROGRAM FOR AT-RISK BENEFICIARIES.—

(A) AUTHORITY TO ESTABLISH.—A PDP sponsor may establish a drug management program for at-risk beneficiaries under which, subject to subparagraph (B), the PDP sponsor may, in the case of an at-risk beneficiary for prescription drug abuse who is an enrollee in a prescription drug plan of such PDP sponsor, limit such beneficiary's access to coverage for frequently abused drugs under such plan to frequently abused drugs that are prescribed for such beneficiary by one or more prescribers selected under subparagraph (D), and dispensed for such beneficiary by one or more pharmacies selected under such subparagraph.

(B) REQUIREMENT FOR NOTICES.—

(i) IN GENERAL.—A PDP sponsor may not limit the access of an at-risk beneficiary for prescription drug abuse to coverage for frequently abused drugs under a prescription drug plan until such sponsor—

(I) provides to the beneficiary an initial notice described in clause (ii) and a second notice described in clause (iii); and

(II) verifies with the providers of the beneficiary that the beneficiary is an at-risk beneficiary for prescription drug abuse.

(ii) INITIAL NOTICE.—An initial notice described in this clause is a notice that provides to the beneficiary—

(I) notice that the PDP sponsor has identified the beneficiary as potentially being an at-risk beneficiary for prescription drug abuse;

(II) information describing all State and Federal public health resources that are designed to address prescription drug abuse to which the beneficiary has access, including mental health services and other counseling services;

(III) notice of, and information about, the right of the beneficiary to appeal such identification under subsection (h) and the option of an automatic escalation to external review;

(IV) a request for the beneficiary to submit to the PDP sponsor preferences for which prescribers and pharmacies the beneficiary would prefer the PDP sponsor to select under subparagraph (D) in the case that the beneficiary is identified as an at-risk beneficiary for prescription drug abuse as described in clause (iii)(I);

(V) an explanation of the meaning and consequences of the identification of the beneficiary as potentially being an at-risk beneficiary for prescription drug abuse, including an explanation of the drug management program established by the PDP sponsor pursuant to subparagraph (A);

(VI) clear instructions that explain how the beneficiary can contact the PDP sponsor in order to submit to the PDP sponsor the preferences described in subclause (IV) and any other communications relating to the drug management program for at-risk beneficiaries established by the PDP sponsor; and

(VII) contact information for other organizations that can provide the beneficiary with assistance regarding such drug management program (similar to the information provided by the Secretary in other standardized notices provided to part D eligible individuals enrolled in prescription drug plans under this part).

(iii) SECOND NOTICE.—A second notice described in this clause is a notice that provides to the beneficiary notice—

(I) that the PDP sponsor has identified the beneficiary as an at-risk beneficiary for prescription drug abuse;

(II) that such beneficiary is subject to the requirements of the drug management program for at-risk beneficiaries established by such PDP sponsor for such plan;

(III) of the prescriber (or prescribers) and pharmacy (or pharmacies) selected for such individual under subparagraph (D);

(IV) of, and information about, the beneficiary's right to appeal such identification under subsection (h) and the option of an automatic escalation to external review;

(V) that the beneficiary can, in the case that the beneficiary has not previously submitted to the PDP sponsor preferences for which prescribers and pharmacies the beneficiary would prefer the PDP sponsor select under subparagraph (D), submit such preferences to the PDP sponsor; and

(VI) that includes clear instructions that explain how the beneficiary can contact the PDP sponsor.

(iv) TIMING OF NOTICES.—

(I) IN GENERAL.—Subject to subclause (II), a second notice described in clause (iii) shall be provided to the beneficiary on a date that is not less than 30 days after an initial notice described in clause (ii) is provided to the beneficiary.

(II) EXCEPTION.—In the case that the PDP sponsor, in conjunction with the Secretary, determines that concerns identified through rulemaking by the Secretary regarding the health or safety of the beneficiary or regarding significant drug diversion activities require the PDP sponsor to provide a second notice described in clause (iii) to the beneficiary on a date that is earlier than the date described in subclause (I), the PDP sponsor may provide such second notice on such earlier date.

(C) AT-RISK BENEFICIARY FOR PRESCRIPTION DRUG ABUSE.—

(i) IN GENERAL.—For purposes of this paragraph, the term "at-risk beneficiary for prescription drug abuse" means a part D eligible individual who is not an exempted individual described in clause (ii) and—

(I) who is identified as such an at-risk beneficiary through the use of clinical guidelines that indicate misuse or abuse of prescription drugs described in subparagraph (G) and that are developed by the Secretary in consultation with PDP sponsors and other stakeholders, including individuals entitled to benefits under part A or enrolled under part B, advocacy groups representing such individuals, physicians, pharmacists, and other clinicians, retail pharmacies, plan sponsors, entities delegated by plan sponsors, and biopharmaceutical manufacturers; or

(II) with respect to whom the PDP sponsor of a prescription drug plan, upon enrolling such individual in such plan, received notice from the Secretary that such individual was identified under this paragraph to be an at-risk beneficiary for prescription drug abuse under the prescription drug plan in which such individual was most recently previously enrolled and such identification has not been terminated under subparagraph (F).

(ii) EXEMPTED INDIVIDUAL DESCRIBED.—An exempted individual described in this clause is an individual who—

(I) receives hospice care under this title;

(II) is a resident of a long-term care facility, of a facility described in section 1905(d), or of another facility for which frequently abused drugs are dispensed for residents through a contract with a single pharmacy; or

(III) the Secretary elects to treat as an exempted individual for purposes of clause (i).

(iii) PROGRAM SIZE.—The Secretary shall establish policies, including the guidelines developed under clause (i)(I) and the exemptions under clause (ii)(III), to ensure that the population of enrollees in a drug management program for at-risk beneficiaries operated by a prescription drug plan can be effectively managed by such plans.

(iv) CLINICAL CONTACT.—With respect to each at-risk beneficiary for prescription drug abuse enrolled in a prescription drug plan offered by a PDP sponsor, the PDP sponsor shall contact the beneficiary's providers who have prescribed frequently abused drugs regarding whether prescribed medications are appropriate for such beneficiary's medical conditions.

(D) SELECTION OF PRESCRIBERS AND PHARMACIES.—

(i) IN GENERAL.—With respect to each at-risk beneficiary for prescription drug abuse enrolled in a prescription drug plan offered by such sponsor, a PDP sponsor shall, based on the preferences submitted to the PDP sponsor by the beneficiary pursuant to clauses (ii)(IV) and (iii)(V) of subparagraph (B) (except as otherwise provided in this subparagraph) select—

(I) one, or, if the PDP sponsor reasonably determines it necessary to provide the beneficiary with reasonable access under clause (ii), more than one, individual who is authorized to prescribe frequently abused drugs (referred to in this paragraph as a "prescriber") who may write prescriptions for such drugs for such beneficiary; and

(II) one, or, if the PDP sponsor reasonably determines it necessary to provide the beneficiary with reasonable access under clause (ii), more than one, pharmacy that may dispense such drugs to such beneficiary.

For purposes of subclause (II), in the case of a pharmacy that has multiple locations that share real-time electronic data, all such locations of the pharmacy shall collectively be treated as one pharmacy.

(ii) REASONABLE ACCESS.—In making the selections under this subparagraph—

(I) a PDP sponsor shall ensure that the beneficiary continues to have reasonable access to frequently abused drugs (as defined in subparagraph (G)), taking into account geographic location, beneficiary preference, impact on costsharing, and reasonable travel time; and

(II) a PDP sponsor shall ensure such access (including access to prescribers and pharmacies with respect to frequently abused drugs) in the case of individuals with multiple residences, in the case of natural disasters and similar situations, and in the case of the provision of emergency services.

(iii) BENEFICIARY PREFERENCES.—If an at-risk beneficiary for prescription drug abuse submits preferences for which in-network prescribers and pharmacies the beneficiary would prefer the PDP sponsor select in response to a notice under subparagraph (B), the PDP sponsor shall—

(I) review such preferences;

(II) select or change the selection of prescribers and pharmacies for the beneficiary based on such preferences; and

(III) inform the beneficiary of such selection or change of selection.

(iv) EXCEPTION REGARDING BENEFICIARY PREFERENCES.—In the case that the PDP sponsor determines that a change to the selection of prescriber or pharmacy under clause (iii)(II) by the PDP sponsor is contributing or would contribute to prescription drug abuse or drug diversion by the beneficiary, the PDP sponsor may change the selection of prescriber or pharmacy for the beneficiary without regard to the preferences of the beneficiary described in clause (iii). If the PDP sponsor changes the selection pursuant to the preceding sentence, the PDP sponsor shall provide the beneficiary with—

(I) at least 30 days written notice of the change of selection; and

(II) a rationale for the change.

(v) CONFIRMATION.—Before selecting a prescriber or pharmacy under this subparagraph, a PDP sponsor must notify the prescriber and pharmacy that the beneficiary involved has been identified for inclusion in the drug management program for at-risk beneficiaries and that the prescriber and pharmacy has been selected as the beneficiary's designated prescriber and pharmacy.

(E) TERMINATIONS AND APPEALS.—The identification of an individual as an at-risk beneficiary for prescription drug abuse under this paragraph, a coverage determination made under a drug management program for at-risk beneficiaries, the selection of prescriber or pharmacy under subparagraph (D), and information to be shared under subparagraph (I), with respect to such individual, shall be subject to reconsideration and appeal under subsection (h) and the option of an automatic escalation to external review to the extent provided by the Secretary.

(F) TERMINATION OF IDENTIFICATION.—

(i) IN GENERAL.—The Secretary shall develop standards for the termination of identification of an individual as an at-risk beneficiary for prescription drug abuse under this paragraph. Under such standards such identification shall terminate as of the earlier of—

(I) the date the individual demonstrates that the individual is no longer likely, in the absence of the restrictions under this paragraph, to be an at-risk beneficiary for prescription drug abuse described in subparagraph (C)(i); and

(II) the end of such maximum period of identification as the Secretary may specify.

(ii) RULE OF CONSTRUCTION.—Nothing in clause (i) shall be construed as preventing a plan from identifying an individual as an at-risk beneficiary for prescription drug abuse under subparagraph (C)(i) after such termination on the basis of additional information on drug use occurring after the date of notice of such termination.

(G) FREQUENTLY ABUSED DRUG.—For purposes of this subsection, the term "frequently abused drug" means a drug that is a controlled substance that the Secretary determines to be frequently abused or diverted.

(H) DATA DISCLOSURE.—

(i) DATA ON DECISION TO IMPOSE LIMITATION.—In the case of an at-risk beneficiary for prescription drug abuse (or an individual who is a potentially at-risk beneficiary for prescription drug abuse) whose access to coverage for frequently abused drugs under a prescription drug plan has been limited by a PDP sponsor under this paragraph, the Secretary shall establish rules and procedures to require the PDP sponsor to disclose data, including any necessary individually identifiable health information, in a form and manner specified by the Secretary, about the decision to impose such limitations and the limitations imposed by the sponsor under this part.

(ii) DATA TO REDUCE FRAUD, ABUSE, AND WASTE.— The Secretary shall establish rules and procedures to require PDP sponsors operating a drug management program for at-risk beneficiaries under this paragraph to provide the Secretary with such data as the Secretary determines appropriate for purposes of identifying patterns of prescription drug utilization for plan enrollees that are outside normal patterns and that may indicate fraudulent, medically unnecessary, or unsafe use.

(I) SHARING OF INFORMATION FOR SUBSEQUENT PLAN ENROLLMENTS.—The Secretary shall establish procedures under which PDP sponsors who offer prescription drug plans shall share information with respect to individuals who are at-risk beneficiaries for prescription drug abuse (or individuals who are potentially at-risk beneficiaries for prescription drug abuse) and enrolled in a prescription drug plan and who subsequently disenroll from such plan and enroll in another prescription drug plan offered by another PDP sponsor.

(J) PRIVACY ISSUES.—Prior to the implementation of the rules and procedures under this paragraph, the Secretary shall clarify privacy requirements, including requirements under the regulations promulgated pursuant to section 264(c) of the Health Insurance Portability and Accountability Act of 1996 (42 U.S.C. 1320d–2 note), related to the sharing of data under subparagraphs (H) and (I) by PDP sponsors. Such clarification shall provide that the sharing of such data shall be considered to be protected health information in accordance with the requirements of the regulations promulgated pursuant to such section 264(c).

(K) EDUCATION.—The Secretary shall provide education to enrollees in prescription drug plans of PDP sponsors and providers regarding the drug management program for at-risk beneficiaries described in this paragraph, including education—

(i) provided by Medicare administrative contractors through the improper payment outreach and education program described in section 1874A(h); and

(ii) through current education efforts (such as State health insurance assistance programs described in subsection (a)(1)(A) of section 119 of the Medicare Improvements for Patients and Providers Act of 2008 (42 U.S.C. 1395b–3 note)) and materials directed toward such enrollees.

(L) APPLICATION UNDER MA–PD PLANS.—Pursuant to section 1860D–21(c)(1), the provisions of this paragraph apply under part D to

MA organizations offering MA–PD plans to MA eligible individuals in the same manner as such provisions apply under this part to a PDP sponsor offering a prescription drug plan to a part D eligible individual.

(M) CMS COMPLIANCE REVIEW.—The Secretary shall ensure that existing plan sponsor compliance reviews and audit processes include the drug management programs for at-risk beneficiaries under this paragraph, including appeals processes under such programs.

(6) UTILIZATION MANAGEMENT TOOL TO PREVENT DRUG ABUSE.—

(A) IN GENERAL.—A tool described in this paragraph is any of the following:

(i) A utilization tool designed to prevent the abuse of frequently abused drugs by individuals and to prevent the diversion of such drugs at pharmacies.

(ii) Retrospective utilization review to identify—

(I) individuals that receive frequently abused drugs at a frequency or in amounts that are not clinically appropriate; and

(II) providers of services or suppliers that may facilitate the abuse or diversion of frequently abused drugs by beneficiaries.

(iii) Consultation with the contractor described in subparagraph (B) to verify if an individual enrolling in a prescription drug plan offered by a PDP sponsor has been previously identified by another PDP sponsor as an individual described in clause (ii)(I).

(B) REPORTING.—A PDP sponsor offering a prescription drug plan (and an MA organization offering an MA–PD plan) in a State shall submit to the Secretary and the Medicare drug integrity contractor with which the Secretary has entered into a contract under section 1893 with respect to such State a report, on a monthly basis, containing information on—

(i) any provider of services or supplier described in subparagraph (A)(ii)(II) that is identified by such plan sponsor (or organization) during the 30-day period before such report is submitted; and

(ii) the name and prescription records of individuals described in paragraph (5)(C).

(C) CMS COMPLIANCE REVIEW.—The Secretary shall ensure that plan sponsor compliance reviews and program audits biennially include a certification that utilization management tools under this paragraph are in compliance with the requirements for such tools.

(6) PROVIDING PRESCRIPTION DRUG PLANS WITH PARTS A AND B CLAIMS DATA TO PROMOTE THE APPROPRIATE USE OF MEDICATIONS AND IMPROVE HEALTH OUTCOMES.—

(A) PROCESS.—Subject to subparagraph (B), the Secretary shall establish a process under which a PDP sponsor of a prescription drug plan may submit a request for the Secretary to provide the sponsor, on a periodic basis and in an electronic format, beginning in plan year 2020, data described in subparagraph (D) with respect to enrollees in such plan. Such data shall be provided without regard to whether such enrollees are described in clause (ii) of paragraph (2)(A).

(B) PURPOSES.—A PDP sponsor may use the data provided to the sponsor pursuant to subparagraph (A) for any of the following purposes:

(i) To optimize therapeutic outcomes through improved medication use, as such phrase is used in clause (i) of paragraph (2)(A).

(ii) To improving care coordination so as to prevent adverse health outcomes, such as preventable emergency department visits and hospital readmissions.

(iii) For any other purpose determined appropriate by the Secretary.

(C) LIMITATIONS ON DATA USE.—A PDP sponsor shall not use data provided to the sponsor pursuant to subparagraph (A) for any of the following purposes:

(i) To inform coverage determinations under this part.

(ii) To conduct retroactive reviews of medically accepted indications determinations.

(iii) To facilitate enrollment changes to a different prescription drug plan or an MA–PD plan offered by the same parent organization.

(iv) To inform marketing of benefits.

(v) For any other purpose that the Secretary determines is necessary to include in order to protect the identity of individuals entitled to, or enrolled for, benefits under this title and to protect the security of personal health information.

(D) DATA DESCRIBED.—The data described in this clause are standardized extracts (as determined by the Secretary) of claims data under parts A and B for items and services furnished under such parts for time periods specified by the Secretary. Such data shall include data as current as practicable.

(d) CONSUMER SATISFACTION SURVEYS.—In order to provide for comparative information under section 1860D–1(c)(3)(A)(v), the Secretary shall conduct consumer satisfaction surveys with respect to PDP sponsors and prescription drug plans in a manner similar to the manner such surveys are conducted for MA organizations and MA plans under part C.

(e) ELECTRONIC PRESCRIPTION PROGRAM.—

(1) APPLICATION OF STANDARDS.—As of such date as the Secretary may specify, but not later than 1 year after the date of promulgation of final standards under paragraph (4)(D), prescriptions and other information described in paragraph (2)(A) for covered part D drugs prescribed for part D eligible individuals that are transmitted electronically shall be transmitted only in accordance with such standards under an electronic prescription drug program that meets the requirements of paragraph (2).

(2) PROGRAM REQUIREMENTS.—Consistent with uniform standards established under paragraph (3)—

(A) PROVISION OF INFORMATION TO PRESCRIBING HEALTH CARE PROFESSIONAL AND DISPENSING PHARMACIES AND PHARMACISTS.—An electronic prescription drug program shall provide for the electronic transmittal to the prescribing health care professional and to the dispensing pharmacy and pharmacist of the prescription and information on eligibility and benefits (including the drugs included in the applicable formulary, any tiered formulary structure, and any requirements for prior authorization) and of the following information with respect to the prescribing and dispensing of a covered part D drug:

(i) Information on the drug being prescribed or dispensed and other drugs listed on the medication history, including information on drug-drug interactions, warnings or cautions, and, when indicated, dosage adjustments.

(ii) Information on the availability of lower cost, therapeutically appropriate alternatives (if any) for the drug prescribed.

(B) APPLICATION TO MEDICAL HISTORY INFORMATION.—Effective on and after such date as the Secretary specifies and after the establishment of appropriate standards to carry out this subparagraph, the program shall provide for the electronic transmittal in a manner similar to the manner under subparagraph (A) of information that relates to the medical history concerning the individual and related to a covered part D drug being prescribed or dispensed, upon request of the professional or pharmacist involved.

(C) LIMITATIONS.—Information shall only be disclosed under subparagraph (A) or (B) if the disclosure of such information is permitted under the Federal regulations (concerning the privacy of individually identifiable health information) promulgated under section 264(c) of the Health Insurance Portability and Accountability Act of 1996.

(D) TIMING.—To the extent feasible, the information exchanged under this paragraph shall be on an interactive, real-time basis.

(3) STANDARDS.—

(A) IN GENERAL.—The Secretary shall provide consistent with this subsection for the promulgation of uniform standards relating to the requirements for electronic prescription drug programs under paragraph (2).

(B) OBJECTIVES.—Such standards shall be consistent with the objectives of improving—

(i) patient safety;

(ii) the quality of care provided to patients; and

(iii) efficiencies, including cost savings, in the delivery of care.

(C) DESIGN CRITERIA.—Such standards shall—

(i) be designed so that, to the extent practicable, the standards do not impose an undue administrative burden on prescribing health care professionals and dispensing pharmacies and pharmacists;

(ii) be compatible with standards established under part C of title XI, standards established under subsection (b)(2)(B)(i), and with general health information technology standards; and

(iii) be designed so that they permit electronic exchange of drug labeling and drug listing information maintained by the Food and Drug Administration and the National Library of Medicine.

(D) PERMITTING USE OF APPROPRIATE MESSAGING.—Such standards shall allow for the messaging of information only if it relates to the appropriate prescribing of drugs, including quality assurance measures and systems referred to in subsection (c)(1)(B).

(E) PERMITTING PATIENT DESIGNATION OF DISPENSING PHARMACY.—

(i) IN GENERAL.—Consistent with clause (ii), such standards shall permit a part D eligible individual to designate a particular pharmacy to dispense a prescribed drug.

(ii) NO CHANGE IN BENEFITS.—Clause (i) shall not be construed as affecting—

(I) the access required to be provided to pharmacies by a prescription drug plan; or

(II) the application of any differences in benefits or payments under such a plan based on the pharmacy dispensing a covered part D drug.

(4) DEVELOPMENT, PROMULGATION, AND MODIFICATION OF STANDARDS.—

(A) INITIAL STANDARDS.—Not later than September 1, 2005, the Secretary shall develop, adopt, recognize, or modify initial uniform standards relating to the requirements for electronic prescription drug programs described in paragraph (2) taking into consideration the recommendations (if any) from the National Committee on Vital and Health Statistics (as established under section 306(k) of the Public Health Service Act (42 U.S.C. 242k(k))) under subparagraph (B).

(B) ROLE OF NCVHS.—The National Committee on Vital and Health Statistics shall develop recommendations for uniform standards relating to such requirements in consultation with the following:

(i) Standard setting organizations (as defined in section 1171(8))

(ii) Practicing physicians.

(iii) Hospitals.

(iv) Pharmacies.

(v) Practicing pharmacists.

(vi) Pharmacy benefit managers.

(vii) State boards of pharmacy.

(viii) State boards of medicine.

(ix) Experts on electronic prescribing.

(x) Other appropriate Federal agencies.

(C) PILOT PROJECT TO TEST INITIAL STANDARDS.—

(i) IN GENERAL.—During the 1-year period that begins on January 1, 2006, the Secretary shall conduct a pilot project to test the initial standards developed under subparagraph (A) prior to the promulgation of the final uniform standards under subparagraph (D) in order to provide for the efficient implementation of the requirements described in paragraph (2).

(ii) EXCEPTION.—Pilot testing of standards is not required under clause (i) where there already is adequate industry experience with such standards, as determined by the Secretary after consultation with effected standard setting organizations and industry users.

(iii) VOLUNTARY PARTICIPATION OF PHYSICIANS AND PHARMACIES.—In order to conduct the pilot project under clause (i), the Secretary shall enter into agreements with physicians, physician groups, pharmacies, hospitals, PDP sponsors, MA organizations, and other appropriate entities under which health care professionals electronically transmit prescriptions to dispensing pharmacies and pharmacists in accordance with such standards.

(iv) EVALUATION AND REPORT.—

(I) EVALUATION.—The Secretary shall conduct an evaluation of the pilot project conducted under clause (i).

(II) REPORT TO CONGRESS.—Not later than April 1, 2007, the Secretary shall submit to Congress a report on the evaluation conducted under subclause (I).

(D) FINAL STANDARDS.—Based upon the evaluation of the pilot project under subparagraph (C)(iv)(I) and not later than April 1, 2008, the Secretary shall promulgate uniform standards relating to the requirements described in paragraph (2).

(5) RELATION TO STATE LAWS.—The standards promulgated under this subsection shall supersede any State law or regulation that—

(A) is contrary to the standards or restricts the ability to carry out this part; and

(B) pertains to the electronic transmission of medication history and of information on eligibility, benefits, and prescriptions with respect to covered part D drugs under this part.

(6) ESTABLISHMENT OF SAFE HARBOR.—The Secretary, in consultation with the Attorney General, shall promulgate regulations that provide for a safe harbor from sanctions under paragraphs (1) and (2) of section 1128B(b) and an exception to the prohibition under subsection (a)(1) of section 1877 with respect to the provision of nonmonetary remuneration (in the form of hardware, software, or information technology and training services) necessary and used solely to receive and transmit electronic prescription information in accordance with the standards promulgated under this subsection—

(A) in the case of a hospital, by the hospital to members of its medical staff;

(B) in the case of a group practice (as defined in section 1877(h)(4)), by the practice to prescribing health care professionals who are members of such practice; and

(C) in the case of a PDP sponsor or MA organization, by the sponsor or organization to pharmacists and pharmacies participating in the network of such sponsor or organization, and to prescribing health care professionals.

(f) GRIEVANCE MECHANISM.—Each PDP sponsor shall provide meaningful procedures for hearing and resolving grievances between the sponsor (including any entity or individual through which the sponsor provides covered benefits) and enrollees with prescription drug plans of the sponsor under this part in accordance with section 1852(f).

(g) COVERAGE DETERMINATIONS AND RECONSIDERATIONS.—

(1) APPLICATION OF COVERAGE DETERMINATION AND RECONSIDERATION PROVISIONS.—A PDP sponsor shall meet the requirements of paragraphs (1) through (3) of section 1852(g) with respect to covered benefits under the prescription drug plan it offers under this part in the same manner as such requirements apply to an MA organization with respect to benefits it offers under an MA plan under part C.

(2) REQUEST FOR A DETERMINATION FOR THE TREATMENT OF TIERED FORMULARY DRUG.—In the case of a prescription drug plan offered by a PDP sponsor that provides for tiered costsharing for drugs included within a formulary and provides lower cost-sharing for preferred drugs included within the formulary, a part D eligible individual who is enrolled in the plan may request an exception to the tiered cost-sharing structure. Under such an exception, a nonpreferred drug could be covered under the terms applicable for preferred drugs if the prescribing physician determines that the preferred drug for treatment of the same condition either would not be as effective for the individual or would have adverse effects for the individual or both. A PDP sponsor shall have an exceptions process under this paragraph consistent with guidelines established by the Secretary for making a determination with respect to such a request. Denial of such an exception shall be treated as a coverage denial for purposes of applying subsection (h).

(h) APPEALS.—

(1) IN GENERAL.—Subject to paragraph (2), a PDP sponsor shall meet the requirements of paragraphs (4) and (5) of section 1852(g) with respect to benefits (including a determination related to the application of tiered cost-sharing described in subsection (g)(2)) in a manner similar (as determined by the Secretary) to the manner such requirements apply to an MA organization with respect to benefits under the original medicare fee-for-service program option it offers under an MA plan under part C. In

applying this paragraph only the part D eligible individual shall be entitled to bring such an appeal.

(2) LIMITATION IN CASES ON NONFORMULARY DETERMINATIONS.—A part D eligible individual who is enrolled in a prescription drug plan offered by a PDP sponsor may appeal under paragraph (1) a determination not to provide for coverage of a covered part D drug that is not on the formulary under the plan only if the prescribing physician determines that all covered part D drugs on any tier of the formulary for treatment of the same condition would not be as effective for the individual as the nonformulary drug, would have adverse effects for the individual, or both.

(3) TREATMENT OF NONFORMULARY DETERMINATIONS.—If a PDP sponsor determines that a plan provides coverage for a covered part D drug that is not on the formulary of the plan, the drug shall be treated as being included on the formulary for purposes of section 1860D–2(b)(4)(C)(i).

(i) PRIVACY, CONFIDENTIALITY, AND ACCURACY OF ENROLLEE RECORDS.—The provisions of section 1852(h) shall apply to a PDP sponsor and prescription drug plan in the same manner as it applies to an MA organization and an MA plan.

(j) TREATMENT OF ACCREDITATION.—Subparagraph (A) of section 1852(e)(4) (relating to treatment of accreditation) shall apply to a PDP sponsor under this part with respect to the following requirements, in the same manner as it applies to an MA organization with respect to the requirements in subparagraph (B) (other than clause (vii) thereof) of such section:

(1) Subsection (b) of this section (relating to access to covered part D drugs).

(2) Subsection (c) of this section (including quality assurance and medication therapy management).

(3) Subsection (i) of this section (relating to confidentiality and accuracy of enrollee records).

(k) PUBLIC DISCLOSURE OF PHARMACEUTICAL PRICES FOR EQUIVALENT DRUGS.—

(1) IN GENERAL.—A PDP sponsor offering a prescription drug plan shall provide that each pharmacy that dispenses a covered part D drug shall inform an enrollee of any differential between the price of the drug to the enrollee and the price of the lowest priced generic covered part D drug under the plan that is therapeutically equivalent and bioequivalent and available at such pharmacy.

(2) TIMING OF NOTICE.—

(A) IN GENERAL.—Subject to subparagraph (B), the information under paragraph (1) shall be provided at the time of purchase of the drug involved, or, in the case of dispensing by mail order, at the time of delivery of such drug.

(B) WAIVER.—The Secretary may waive subparagraph (A) in such circumstances as the Secretary may specify.

(l) REQUIREMENTS WITH RESPECT TO SALES AND MARKETING ACTIVITIES.—The following provisions shall apply to a PDP sponsor (and the agents, brokers, and other third parties representing such sponsor) in the same manner as such provisions apply to a Medicare Advantage organization (and the agents, brokers, and other third parties representing such organization):

(1) The prohibition under section 1851(h)(4)(C) on conducting activities described in section 1851(j)(1).

(2) The requirement under section 1851(h)(4)(D) to conduct activities described in section 1851(j)(2) in accordance with the limitations established under such subsection.

(3) The inclusion of the plan type in the plan name under section 1851(h)(6).

(4) The requirements regarding the appointment of agents and brokers and compliance with State information requests under subparagraphs (A) and (B), respectively, of section 1851(h)(7).

(m) PROGRAM INTEGRITY TRANSPARENCY MEASURES.—For pro- gram integrity transparency measures applied with respect to pre- scription drug plan and MA plans, see section 1859(i).

EXCHANGE OF LETTERS WITH ADDITIONAL COMMITTEES OF REFERRAL

GREG WALDEN, OREGON
CHAIRMAN

FRANK PALLONE, JR., NEW JERSEY
RANKING MEMBER

ONE HUNDRED FIFTEENTH CONGRESS

**Congress of the United States**

**House of Representatives**

COMMITTEE ON ENERGY AND COMMERCE

2125 RAYBURN HOUSE OFFICE BUILDING
WASHINGTON, DC 20515-6115

Majority (202) 225-2927
Minority (202) 225-3641

June 7, 2018

The Honorable Kevin Brady
Chairman
Committee on Ways and Means
1102 Longworth House Office Building
Washington, DC 20515

Dear Chairman Brady:

On May 9 and 17, 2018, the Committee on Energy and Commerce ordered favorably reported over 50 bills to address the opioid epidemic facing communities across our nation. Several of the bills were also referred to the Committee on Ways and Means.

I ask that the Committee on Ways and Means not insist on its referral of the following bills so that they may be scheduled for consideration by the Majority Leader:

- **H.R. 1925**, At-Risk Youth Medicaid Protection Act of 2017;
- **H.R. 3331**, To amend title XI of the Social Security Act to promote testing of incentive payments for behavioral health providers for adoption and use of certified electronic health record technology;
- **H.R. 3528**, Every Prescription Conveyed Securely Act;
- **H.R. 4841**, Standardizing Electronic Prior Authorization for Safe Prescribing Act of 2018;
- **H.R. 5582**, Abuse Deterrent Access Act of 2018;
- **H.R. 5590**, Opioid Addiction Action Plan Act;
- **H.R. 5603**, Access to Telehealth Services for Opioid Use Disorder;

The Honorable Kevin Brady
Page 2

- **H.R. 5605**, Advancing High Quality Treatment for Opioid Use Disorders in Medicare Act;
- **H.R. 5675**, To amend title XVIII of the Social Security Act to require prescription drug plan sponsors under the Medicare program to establish drug management programs for at-risk beneficiaries;
- **H.R. 5684**, Protecting Seniors from Opioid Abuse Act;
- **H.R. 5685**, Medicare Opioid Safety Education Act;
- **H.R. 5686**, Medicare Clear Health Options in Care for Enrollees (CHOICE) Act;
- **H.R. 5715**, Strengthening Partnerships to Prevent Opioid Abuse Act;
- **H.R. 5716**, Commit to Opioid Medical Prescriber Accountability and Safety for Seniors (COMPASS) Act;
- **H.R. 5796**, Responsible Education Achieves Care and Healthy Outcomes for Users' Treatment (REACH OUT) Act of 2018;
- **H.R. 5798**, Opioid Screening and Chronic Pain Management Alternatives for Seniors Act;
- **H.R. 5804**, Post-Surgical Injections as an Opioid Alternative Act; and
- **H.R. 5809**, Postoperative Opioid Prevention Act of 2018.

This concession in no way affects your jurisdiction over the subject matter of these bills, and it will not serve as precedent for future referrals. In addition, should a conference on the bills be necessary, I would support your request to have the Committee on Ways and Means on the conference committee. Finally, I would be pleased to include this letter and your response in the bill reports and the Congressional Record.

Thank you for your consideration of my request and for the extraordinary cooperation shown by you and your staff over matters of shared jurisdiction. I look forward to further opportunities to work with you this Congress.

Sincerely,

Greg Walden
Chairman

**Congress of the United States**
**U.S. House of Representatives**
COMMITTEE ON WAYS AND MEANS

1102 LONGWORTH HOUSE OFFICE BUILDING
(202) 225-3625
Washington, DC 20515-0348
http://waysandmeans.house.gov



June 8, 2018

The Honorable Greg Walden
Chairman
Committee on Energy and Commerce
2125 Rayburn House Office Building
Washington, DC 20515

Dear Chairman Walden,

Thank you for your letter concerning several bills favorably reported out of the Committee on Energy and Commerce to address the opioid epidemic and which the Committee on Ways and Means was granted an additional referral.

As a result of your having consulted with us on provisions within these bills that fall within the Rule X jurisdiction of the Committee on Ways and Means, I agree to waive formal consideration of the following bills so that they may move expeditiously to the floor:

- **H.R. 1925**, At-Risk Youth Medicaid Protection Act of 2017;
- **H.R. 3331,** To amend title XI of the Social Security Act to promote testing of incentive payments for behavioral health providers for adoption and use of certified electronic health record technology;
- **H.R. 3528**, Every Prescription Conveyed Securely Act;
- **H.R. 4841**, Standardizing Electronic Prior Authorization for Safe Prescribing Act of 2018;
- **H.R. 5582**, Abuse Deterrent Access Act of 2018;
- **H.R. 5590**, Opioid Addiction Action Plan Act;
- **H.R. 5603**, Access to Telehealth Services for Opioid Use Disorder;
- **H.R. 5605**, Advancing High Quality Treatment for Opioid Use Disorders in Medicare Act;

- **H.R. 5675,** To amend title XVIII of the Social Security Act to require prescription drug plan sponsors under the Medicare program to establish drug management programs for at-risk beneficiaries;
- **H.R. 5684,** Protecting Seniors from Opioid Abuse Act;
- **H.R. 5685,** Medicare Opioid Safety Education Act;
- **H.R. 5686,** Medicare Clear Health Options in Care for Enrollees (CHOICE) Act;
- **H.R. 5715,** Strengthening Partnerships to Prevent Opioid Abuse Act;
- **H.R. 5716,** Commit to Opioid Medical Prescriber Accountability and Safety for Seniors (COMPASS) Act;
- **H.R. 5796,** Responsible Education Achieves Care and Healthy Outcomes for Users' Treatment (REACH OUT) Act of 2018;
- **H.R. 5798,** Opioid Screening and Chronic Pain Management Alternatives for Seniors Act;
- **H.R. 5804,** Post-Surgical Injections as an Opioid Alternative Act; and
- **H.R. 5809,** Postoperative Opioid Prevention Act of 2018.

The Committee on Ways and Means takes this action with the mutual understanding that we do not waive any jurisdiction over the subject matter contained in this or similar legislation, and the Committee will be appropriately consulted and involved as the bill or similar legislation moves forward so that we may address any remaining issues that fall within our jurisdiction. The Committee also reserves the right to seek appointment of an appropriate number of conferees to any House-Senate conference involving this or similar legislation and requests your support for such a request.

Finally, I would appreciate your commitment to include this exchange of letters in the bill reports and the Congressional Record.

Sincerely,

Kevin Brady
Chairman

cc: The Honorable Paul Ryan, Speaker
The Honorable Richard E. Neal
The Honorable Frank Pallone
Thomas J. Wickham, Jr., Parliamentarian

O

# INDEX

## A

abuse, 2, 29, 30, 132, 155, 156, 180, 181, 183, 209, 210, 217, 218, 220, 249, 250, 257, 264, 269
access, 15, 29, 38, 39, 40, 45, 63, 69, 75, 80, 85, 102, 108, 109, 120, 132, 142, 155, 164, 165, 166, 170, 195, 209, 219, 243, 247, 251, 252, 253, 254, 256, 257, 259, 261, 262, 265, 267, 273, 277
accreditation, 43, 94, 107, 109, 277
age, vii, 2, 7, 11, 103, 113, 122, 132, 137, 138, 183, 191
agencies, 5, 6, 33, 52, 64, 68, 70, 71, 72, 84, 93, 135, 136, 159, 186, 187, 213, 242, 274
alternative treatments, 19, 146, 199
analgesic, 16, 31, 143, 157, 196, 211
aneurysm, 59, 60, 111, 114
antipsychotic, 12, 139, 192
antipsychotic drugs, 12, 139, 192
appropriations, 18, 23, 145, 150, 198, 206
assessment, 2, 16, 17, 85, 101, 115, 117, 119, 123, 143, 144, 196, 197, 198, 231, 239, 240, 241
authority, 4, 6, 10, 17, 18, 27, 28, 33, 34, 35, 77, 78, 134, 136, 137, 144, 145, 151, 155, 159, 161, 185, 187, 190, 197, 199, 208, 209, 213, 215, 222
avoidance, 28, 154, 208

## B

beneficiaries, vii, 2, 9, 13, 15, 19, 29, 72, 114, 123, 124, 127, 129, 131, 132, 140, 142, 146, 155, 165, 166, 168, 169, 170, 171, 183, 190, 193, 195, 196, 199, 209, 233, 243, 247, 248, 251, 258, 259, 260, 261, 262, 263, 264, 266, 267, 268, 269
benefits, 35, 38, 40, 45, 47, 54, 66, 70, 72, 77, 95, 99, 105, 107, 109, 115, 122, 161, 164, 170, 215, 218, 221, 223, 226, 233, 234, 235, 237, 238, 239, 240, 244, 245, 247, 251, 252, 253, 264, 270, 271, 273, 275, 276
blood, 51, 57, 59, 103, 110, 111, 112, 118, 122
blood clot, 57
blood pressure, 110, 118, 122
body mass index, 110, 113, 118, 122

bone, 61, 101, 105
bone mass, 61, 105
breast cancer, 100
budget deficit, 5, 32, 135, 159, 187, 213

## C

cancer, 103, 104, 110
cancer screening, 110
certification, 62, 89, 93, 99, 110, 169, 270
children, 7, 11, 12, 23, 138, 139, 150, 191, 192, 206
chronic diseases, 123, 258
chronic heart failure, 118
chronic kidney disease, 120
clinical trials, 35, 161, 215, 255
communication, 180, 183, 217, 219, 249
congestive heart failure, 258
controlled substances, 5, 12, 13, 14, 15, 19, 26, 29, 31, 35, 135, 139, 140, 141, 142, 146, 151, 156, 157, 161, 186, 193, 194, 196, 199, 204, 207, 210, 211, 215
coordination, 124, 125, 166, 236, 244, 260, 270
coronary angioplasty, 118
coronary bypass surgery, 117, 118
coronary heart disease, 117
cost, 1, 4, 6, 7, 11, 13, 16, 21, 22, 23, 27, 28, 29, 30, 31, 34, 35, 37, 64, 65, 66, 68, 69, 70, 71, 72, 73, 74, 75, 76, 77, 79, 80, 93, 94, 114, 134, 136, 138, 140, 143, 148, 149, 150, 151, 154, 155, 156, 157, 160, 161, 164, 179, 185, 187, 191, 194, 196, 201, 202, 204, 205, 206, 207, 208, 209, 210, 211, 214, 215, 218, 227, 239, 247, 251, 254, 256, 257, 258, 272, 276
cost saving, 93, 272
counseling, 91, 92, 95, 98, 109, 110, 117, 122, 166, 168, 225, 258, 262

## D

data collection, 27, 154, 208
data set, 12, 139, 192
Department of Health and Human Services, 3, 5, 7, 36, 132, 135, 136, 162, 184, 186, 188, 216, 261
Department of Justice, 27, 151, 207
detection, vii, 2, 100, 103, 104, 109, 110, 112, 114, 115, 258
diabetes, 51, 58, 59, 61, 104, 105, 112, 113, 118, 258
dialysis, 56, 58, 59, 120, 121
diastolic blood pressure, 118
disclosure, 30, 157, 211, 272
discrimination, 30, 157, 211
diseases, 31, 43, 53, 59, 86, 157, 167, 211
disorder, vii, 1, 2, 11, 14, 15, 16, 22, 26, 30, 37, 39, 110, 111, 131, 132, 138, 141, 142, 143, 149, 151, 156, 163, 165, 166, 168, 169, 170, 171, 172, 192, 195, 196, 204, 205, 207, 210
drug abuse, 258, 267, 268
drug interaction, 257, 258, 272
drug therapy, 105, 258
drugs, 5, 12, 13, 14, 16, 17, 27, 28, 29, 31, 34, 35, 40, 46, 47, 50, 56, 62, 63, 84, 85, 89, 91, 98, 104, 106, 125, 126, 135, 139, 140, 141, 143, 144, 154, 155, 156, 157, 160, 161, 166, 169, 186, 192, 194, 197, 198, 208, 209, 210, 211, 214, 215, 251, 252, 253,255, 256, 257, 258, 260, 261, 262, 264, 265, 267, 269, 271, 272, 273, 275, 276, 277

## E

education, 16, 22, 36, 60, 80, 87, 88, 98, 110, 117, 119, 120, 121, 125, 143, 149, 162, 196, 205, 216, 258, 268
educational opportunities, 44

educational services, 120
emergency, 21, 69, 70, 85, 148, 167, 201, 244, 253, 265, 270
employees, 27, 74, 80, 151, 207, 223, 233
employment, 38, 44, 66, 79, 164, 219, 223
employment relationship, 79
end stage renal disease, 247
enforcement, 32, 158, 212
enrollment, 13, 140, 194, 225, 227, 229, 231, 233, 236, 237, 238, 239, 241, 247, 248, 251, 259, 260, 270
epidemic, 3, 5, 126, 128, 132, 134, 184, 186
equipment, 40, 46, 50, 51, 56, 60, 83, 89, 125
evidence, vii, 2, 15, 27, 61, 63, 118, 132, 142, 151, 181, 183, 195, 207, 223, 250, 255
evidence-based practices, 27, 151, 207
exclusion, 11, 125, 139, 180, 192, 249
expenditures, 4, 116, 134, 166, 185, 226

## F

families, 23, 30, 150, 157, 206, 211
family history, 59, 60, 104, 113, 121
federal government, 11, 24, 138, 139, 150, 192, 207
federal law, 26, 151, 207
financial, 18, 52, 68, 97, 145, 198, 222, 223, 224, 234, 237, 245
financial records, 222
fiscal year, 8, 9, 10, 16, 20, 21, 24, 25, 26, 28, 71, 72, 73, 75, 76, 77, 143, 148, 154, 173, 189, 190, 196, 200, 201, 202, 208, 225, 226
Food and Drug Administration, 5, 10, 16, 24, 36, 58, 59, 63, 105, 135, 144, 162, 186, 190, 197, 202, 216, 273
fraud, 2, 30, 132, 156, 180, 181, 183, 210, 217, 218, 220, 249, 250, 257
funding, 13, 15, 22, 87, 121, 140, 142, 149, 193, 195, 205
funds, 12, 28, 29, 87, 139, 154, 155, 193, 209, 248

## G

generic drugs, 28, 154, 209
gestational diabetes, 113
glaucoma, 59, 109, 111
glucose, 51, 112, 113
glucose tolerance, 113
governments, 33, 159, 213
grant programs, 33, 159, 213
grants, 5, 15, 21, 22, 23, 27, 135, 143, 148, 149, 150, 151, 186, 196, 201, 204, 205, 206, 207
guidance, 26, 27, 29, 30, 63, 84, 124, 151, 154, 155, 156, 181, 204, 207, 208, 209, 210, 218, 230, 250
guidelines, 88, 95, 98, 99, 117, 119, 120, 121, 122, 123, 171, 172, 260, 264, 276

## H

health, 6, 7, 8, 11, 14, 15, 18, 21, 23, 26, 30, 33, 43, 44, 45, 46, 47, 49, 50, 52, 53, 54, 56, 57, 60, 61, 62, 63, 64, 68, 70, 71, 72, 73, 74, 78, 79, 80, 81, 82, 83, 84, 85, 86, 87, 88, 90, 91, 93, 96, 97, 99, 101, 102, 106, 107, 108, 109, 110, 111, 113, 115,121, 122, 123, 124, 127, 129, 136, 138, 141, 142, 145, 148, 150, 151, 157, 160, 167, 168, 169, 170, 181, 187, 189, 191, 192, 194, 195, 198, 199, 201, 204, 206, 207, 211, 214, 221, 223, 225, 227, 230, 232, 234, 236, 237, 238, 244, 245, 247, 250, 255, 263, 267, 268, 270, 271, 272, 273, 274, 275
health care, 14, 21, 23, 26, 30, 43, 74, 81, 85, 86, 88, 106, 107, 108, 111, 113, 115,

123, 141, 148, 150, 151, 157, 168, 169, 170, 194, 201, 206, 207, 211, 230, 255, 271, 273, 274, 275
health care professionals, 14, 115, 141, 194, 273, 274, 275
health education, 122
health effects, 23, 150, 206
health information, 124, 181, 250, 267, 268, 271, 272, 273
health insurance, 225, 268
health promotion, 110
health risks, 122
health services, 49, 56, 64, 78, 84, 85, 86, 96, 97, 102, 106, 108, 109, 223, 244, 245
health status, 122, 124, 237, 238
healthcare coverage, vii, 2, 131, 183
heart failure, 118
hepatitis, 22, 61, 110, 149, 167, 205
hospice, 26, 63, 80, 91, 92, 93, 94, 95, 96, 151, 207, 264

## I

identification, 82, 113, 262, 263, 264, 266, 267
individuals, 2, 14, 15, 41, 42, 43, 45, 47, 49, 51, 52, 54, 59, 62, 64, 70, 77, 85, 90, 92, 93, 95, 96, 97, 99, 105, 106, 107, 112, 114, 115, 118, 119, 126, 132, 141, 142, 167, 168, 169, 183, 195, 221, 225, 226, 228, 229, 231, 232, 233, 235, 236, 237, 238, 239, 240, 241, 242, 243, 244, 245, 246, 247, 248, 253, 254, 258, 259, 263, 264, 265, 268, 269, 270, 271
industry, 27, 121, 154, 208, 260, 274
infants, 26, 30, 156, 204, 210
inflammatory bowel disease, 104
information exchange, 272
information technology, 275
injections, 16, 31, 128, 143, 157, 196, 211
injury, iv, 56, 111, 123
institutions, 7, 11, 31, 44, 49, 54, 64, 108, 137, 138, 157, 191, 192, 211
integration, 124, 242, 244, 246
integrity, 179, 180, 182, 183, 249, 269, 278
issues, 23, 130, 150, 206

## J

jurisdiction, 55, 128, 129, 130
juveniles, 7, 137, 191

## K

kidney, 56, 60, 120, 121
kinship, 11, 138, 191

## L

labeling, 27, 31, 154, 157, 208, 212, 273
laboratory tests, 60, 110
law enforcement, 182, 250
laws and regulations, 106
legislation, 3, 4, 5, 6, 7, 16, 17, 18, 28, 29, 31, 32, 35, 37, 38, 130, 132, 133, 134, 135, 136, 143, 144, 145, 154, 155, 157, 158, 161, 163, 164, 184, 185, 186, 187, 188, 196, 198, 199, 208, 209, 211, 212, 215, 217, 219
long-term services, 244, 245
long-term services and supports, 244, 245

## M

mammography, 60, 61, 100, 110
management, 9, 15, 16, 19, 35, 36, 58, 59, 84, 91, 104, 105, 109, 110, 111, 118, 119, 120, 122, 124, 127, 129, 142, 143, 146, 161, 162, 166, 170, 171, 190, 195, 196, 199, 216, 223, 224, 240, 251, 256,

257, 258, 259, 260, 261, 262, 263, 264, 266, 267, 268, 269, 270, 277
marketing, 17, 27, 28, 144, 151, 154, 197, 207, 208, 230, 270
materials, 23, 26, 30, 60, 150, 151, 157, 206, 207, 211, 268
matter, iv, 39, 128, 130, 165, 220
measurement, 61, 105, 109, 110, 122
Medicaid, 3, 5, 7, 8, 11, 12, 13, 17, 18, 23, 24, 26, 29, 30, 31, 32, 33, 36, 37, 127, 129, 132, 133, 135, 136, 137, 138, 139, 140, 144, 145, 150, 155, 156, 157, 158, 159, 162, 163, 173, 183, 184, 186, 188, 189, 191, 192, 193, 197, 199, 202, 204, 206, 209, 210, 211, 212, 213, 216, 239, 242, 244, 245, 246
medical, 26, 27, 30, 40, 41, 43, 46, 47, 48, 49, 50, 51, 56, 57, 58, 59, 60, 62, 63, 65, 70, 71, 75, 78, 83, 84, 86, 88, 89, 91, 93, 96, 98, 102, 103, 106, 107, 108, 109, 110, 115, 116, 117, 119, 121, 122, 124, 125, 151, 154, 157, 207, 208, 211, 223, 227, 229, 230, 236, 239, 241, 255, 265, 272, 275
medical assistance, 236, 239, 241
medical care, 86, 93, 121
medical history, 272
medical reason, 78
Medicare, v, vii, 1, 2, 3, 5, 6, 7, 9, 14, 15, 16, 18, 19, 29, 30, 31, 35, 36, 37, 39, 71, 97, 114, 126, 127, 129, 131, 132, 135, 136, 141, 142, 143, 145, 146, 155, 156, 157, 162, 163, 165, 168, 170, 173, 179, 180, 181, 183, 184, 186, 187, 188, 189, 190, 194, 195, 196, 197, 199, 209, 210, 211, 216, 217, 218, 219, 220, 221, 222, 223, 224, 225, 226, 228, 229, 231, 232, 233, 234, 235, 236, 237, 238, 241, 242, 245, 246, 248, 249, 250, 268, 269, 278
Medicare Part D, vii, 2, 14, 15, 19, 30, 132, 141, 142, 146, 156, 183, 194, 196, 199, 210
Medicare system, vii, 2, 132, 183
medication, 13, 14, 15, 29, 36, 132, 140, 141, 142, 155, 162, 166, 167, 172, 194, 195, 196, 209, 216, 251, 257, 258, 259, 260, 270, 272, 275, 277
medicine, 17, 55, 118, 119, 144, 169, 172, 197, 274
mental health, 7, 14, 18, 21, 97, 98, 99, 122, 132, 136, 141, 145, 148, 165, 166, 167, 188, 195, 198, 201, 262
mental health professionals, 21, 97, 148, 201
mental illness, 100, 247
mentally ill persons, 45
misuse, vii, 2, 29, 132, 156, 183, 210, 264

## N

National Institutes of Health, 36, 162, 216
natural disaster, 265
nursing, 40, 42, 44, 46, 47, 48, 49, 50, 52, 63, 66, 67, 69, 76, 78, 80, 81, 82, 84, 87, 89, 91, 94, 100, 106, 108, 125, 244, 260
nursing care, 46, 50, 51, 84, 89, 91, 94
nursing home, 244
nutrition, 59, 109, 110, 111, 122

## O

occupational therapy, 46, 50, 56, 79, 89, 91, 97
opioid misuse, vii, 2, 132, 183
opioid prescriptions, vii, 1, 2, 12, 16, 37, 39, 110, 111, 132, 139, 143, 183, 192, 196, 220
opioid use disorder, v, vii, 1, 2, 9, 11, 14, 16, 22, 26, 37, 39, 110, 111, 127, 129, 131, 132, 138, 141, 142, 143, 149, 151, 163, 165, 166, 167, 168, 169, 170, 171, 172, 189, 190, 192, 195, 196, 205, 207

opioids, vii, 2, 12, 16, 19, 21, 22, 28, 30, 111, 132, 139, 143, 146, 148, 149, 154, 156, 182, 183, 192, 196, 200, 201, 205, 208, 210, 218, 228
osteoporosis, 50, 100, 101, 105
outpatient, 16, 46, 50, 53, 54, 56, 58, 59, 63, 69, 75, 82, 84, 86, 87, 89, 90, 92, 101, 102, 104, 105, 110, 116, 143, 166, 167, 168, 197
outpatients, 53, 54, 56, 84, 90, 98
oversight, 5, 27, 135, 151, 186, 207
ownership, 68, 74, 106, 108

P

pain, vii, 1, 2, 5, 16, 19, 21, 27, 70, 91, 111, 132, 135, 143, 146, 148, 154, 183, 186, 196, 199, 201, 208
pain management, 16, 19, 21, 143, 146, 148, 196, 199, 201
pain-related conditions, vii, 2, 132, 183
participants, 166, 168, 171, 172, 233
pathology, 46, 50, 56, 89, 91, 101, 102
pathophysiology, 118, 119
penalties, 17, 80, 144, 198, 230, 231, 232
peripheral neuropathy, 61
permit, 14, 29, 34, 35, 141, 156, 160, 161, 195, 210, 215, 220, 227, 252, 253, 255, 256, 260, 273
pharmaceutical, 13, 31, 140, 157, 194, 211, 255
physical activity, 122
physical health, 18, 145, 198
physical therapist, 53, 54, 101
physical therapy, 46, 53, 54, 56, 79, 89, 90, 101
physician involvement, 115
physicians, 41, 47, 52, 53, 55, 56, 57, 58, 65, 70, 79, 80, 83, 84, 89, 90, 91, 97, 99, 110, 115, 121, 167, 234, 248, 254, 256, 260, 264, 274
policy, 7, 11, 136, 138, 188, 191, 192, 234, 239
population, vii, viii, 2, 86, 131, 132, 163, 183, 240, 247, 264
prescription drug abuse, 15, 142, 196, 261, 262, 263, 264, 265, 266, 267, 268
prescription drugs, 12, 57, 139, 192, 247, 258, 264
prevention, 60, 115, 116, 120, 121, 122, 123, 124
primary hyperparathyroidism, 105
professional management, 92
professionals, 21, 121, 122, 148, 204
project, vii, 131, 163, 248, 274, 275
prostate cancer, 58, 103
prosthetic device, 60
psychoactive drug, 23, 150, 206
psychologist, 40, 42, 57, 58, 83, 100
psychosocial support, 132
public health, 22, 34, 53, 54, 149, 160, 205, 214, 262
public interest, 49
public service, 38, 164, 219
pulmonary rehabilitation, 60, 119

Q

quality assurance, 273, 277
quality improvement, 66, 81
quality standards, 104, 105

R

recognition, 65, 75, 254
recommendations, iv, 122, 124, 273, 274
regulations, 28, 29, 30, 44, 48, 50, 54, 57, 60, 61, 64, 65, 66, 69, 73, 74, 75, 79, 81, 82, 85, 86, 87, 89, 90, 98, 101, 105, 114, 154, 155, 157, 169, 181, 208, 209, 211, 222, 223, 230, 237, 238, 244, 248, 250, 268, 272, 275

rehabilitation, 41, 43, 50, 53, 54, 60, 63, 82, 86, 89, 90, 101, 116, 117, 118, 119
rehabilitation program, 60, 116, 117, 118, 119
resources, 242, 260, 262
response, 5, 105, 128, 134, 186, 266
risk, 2, 9, 13, 15, 29, 57, 59, 60, 61, 103, 104, 105, 111, 112, 113, 115, 121, 122, 123, 124, 127, 129, 140, 142, 156, 190, 193, 195, 196, 210, 223, 232, 234, 236, 251, 253, 258, 259, 261, 262, 263, 264, 265, 266, 267, 268, 269
risk assessment, 121, 122, 123, 124
risk factors, 2, 60, 111, 113, 115, 122, 123

## S

safety, 43, 44, 45, 51, 52, 54, 60, 62, 85, 90, 93, 99, 107, 255, 263, 272
Secretary of HHS, 11, 14, 15, 19, 20, 21, 22, 23, 29, 30, 34, 138, 141, 142, 143, 146, 147, 148, 149, 150, 155, 156, 157, 160, 161, 191, 195, 196, 199, 200, 201, 204, 205, 206, 209, 210, 211, 214, 215
services, iv, 11, 14, 15, 16, 22, 33, 39, 40, 41, 42, 43, 44, 45, 46, 47, 48, 49, 50, 52, 53, 54, 55, 56, 57, 58, 59, 60, 61, 62, 63, 64, 65, 66, 67, 68, 69, 70, 71, 72, 73, 74, 75, 76, 77, 78, 79, 80, 81, 82, 83, 84, 85, 86, 87, 88, 89, 90, 91, 92, 93, 94, 95, 96, 97, 98, 99, 100, 101, 102, 104, 105, 106, 107, 108, 109, 110, 111, 113, 114, 115, 116, 117, 118, 119, 120, 121, 122, 124, 125, 126, 132, 139, 141, 142, 143, 149, 159, 165, 166, 167, 168, 169, 170, 171, 172, 180, 181, 182, 192, 195, 196, 205, 213, 218, 222, 223, 227, 228, 229, 230, 234, 235, 237, 239, 240, 242, 243, 244, 245, 248, 249, 258, 259, 260, 262, 265, 269, 271, 275
Social Security, 1, 8, 9, 11, 15, 18, 39, 80, 127, 129, 138, 142, 145, 179, 180, 182, 189, 190, 192, 195, 199
social services, 40, 46, 50, 91, 168
social support, 166
social workers, 97
speech, 46, 50, 51, 56, 79, 89, 91, 101, 102
spending, 2, 5, 6, 7, 10, 11, 12, 13, 14, 15, 16, 17, 18, 19, 20, 21, 22, 23, 24, 26, 27, 28, 29, 30, 31, 32, 132, 135, 136, 137, 138, 139, 140, 141, 142, 143, 144, 145, 146, 147, 148, 149, 150, 151, 152, 153, 154, 155, 156, 157, 158, 167, 183, 186, 187, 188, 189,190, 191, 192, 193, 194, 195, 196, 197, 198, 199, 200, 201, 202, 204, 205, 206, 207, 208, 209, 210, 211, 212, 213
stakeholders, 23, 36, 132, 150, 162, 172, 180, 181, 182, 206, 216, 228, 243, 244, 249, 250, 259, 260, 261, 264
substance abuse, 5, 7, 18, 135, 136, 145, 186, 188, 198
substance use, 5, 11, 13, 14, 21, 26, 30, 33, 132, 135, 138, 140, 141, 147, 148, 156, 157, 159, 186, 191, 193, 195, 201, 204, 210, 211, 214
substance use disorders, 5, 11, 13, 14, 21, 30, 33, 135, 138, 140, 141, 147, 148, 156, 157, 159, 186, 191, 193, 195, 201, 204, 211, 214
supervision, 41, 43, 45, 46, 50, 52, 53, 54, 57, 58, 60, 84, 88, 89, 90, 91, 96, 97, 100, 106, 107, 109, 110, 114, 116, 117, 119, 122
supplier, 41, 51, 77, 124, 125, 126, 181, 228, 230, 249, 269
suppliers, 30, 121, 156, 166, 171, 180, 210, 228, 249, 269

## T

tariff, 38, 164, 218
technical assistance, 16, 143, 196
technical support, 23, 150, 206
technology, 18, 34, 103, 124, 127, 129, 145, 161, 180, 181, 199, 215, 249, 250, 253, 254, 273
testing, 18, 22, 51, 89, 112, 127, 129, 145, 149, 199, 205, 248, 274
therapy, 13, 15, 36, 50, 53, 54, 57, 59, 60, 79, 89, 104, 105, 109, 110, 111, 118, 120, 124, 125, 126, 140, 142, 162, 194, 196, 216, 251, 257, 258, 259, 260, 277
time periods, 271
total revenue, 227
training, 21, 23, 30, 40, 46, 50, 51, 58, 59, 66, 87, 88, 89, 91, 98, 104, 105, 110, 119, 148, 150, 157, 204, 206, 211, 240, 275
training programs, 30, 157, 211
treatment, viii, 2, 5, 7, 11, 13, 14, 15, 18, 22, 28, 29, 33, 40, 41, 43, 45, 46, 47, 49, 53, 55, 59, 84, 85, 86, 97, 98, 100, 106, 107, 108, 111, 112, 113, 115, 116, 117, 119, 122, 131, 132, 135, 136, 138, 140, 141, 142, 145, 149, 154, 155, 159, 163, 165, 166, 167, 168, 169, 170, 171, 172, 186, 188, 191, 194, 195, 198, 205, 208, 209, 214, 256, 257, 276, 277

## U

uniform, 55, 66, 76, 242, 257, 260, 271, 272, 273, 274, 275
United States, 26, 30, 60, 62, 63, 81, 109, 112, 115, 122, 126, 128, 156, 204, 210, 222, 255
updating, 73, 83, 247

## W

waiver, 13, 44, 88, 94, 140, 169, 194
waste, 30, 156, 180, 181, 183, 210, 217, 218, 220, 249, 250, 257, 260
workload, 23, 28, 150, 155, 206, 209